#Lemonadelife

The Book

Yusef Harris

For permission requests, contact: Purpose Publishing via email at contactus@purposepublishing.com.

For speaking engagements, interviews, bulk orders, or promotions contact the author and stay connected at divinecontroller@gmail.com

Printed in the United States of America

Paperback ISBN 978-1-965319-65-9
eBook ISBN 978-1-965319-66-6

Library of Congress Control Number: 2026903039

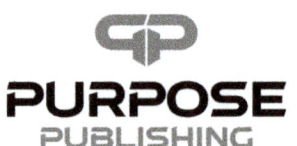

PURPOSE
PUBLISHING

Purpose Publishing LLC.
13194 US Highway 301 South, Suite 417
Riverview, Florida 33578

www.PurposePublishing.com

Dedication

I would like to dedicate this book to my inspiration,
Shakur Ahmed Harris.
"Thank you for showing up right on time. Be the greatest there ever was."
—Love Papi

To my nephew Vincent Vernard Taylor.
"Thank you for being honest, reliable, and true. This world changed in a way I can never get used to after you were murdered and taken from us. Love you, nephew."

To Mr. Brent Flournoy.
"Thank you for caring, thank you for asking questions, and thank you for being willing to help me in my health journey. The conversation we had in the barbershop was the catalyst for getting me started on this book. Thank you for the motivation."

Contents

Foreword

In medicine, we often say that data tells the story. But the truth is, the patients do.

Statistics can reveal disparities, charts can expose trends, and peer-reviewed journals can confirm what many communities already know—but none of these carry the weight of lived experience. *#LemonadeLife* does.

Yusef Harris invites us into the intimate spaces where healthcare decisions are made, delayed, dismissed, or denied. His story is not simply about illness, survival, or recovery. It is about navigation. Navigation through a healthcare system that is too often inequitable, opaque, and shaped by assumptions that place patients who are Black at a disadvantage long before they ever see a physician.

As an educator and nurse practitioner, I recognize in these pages what research has repeatedly confirmed: racial bias in medicine is not always loud or intentional, but it is persistent—and deadly. From delayed diagnoses to unequal access to specialty care, from being unheard to being undertreated, the experiences described in *#LemonadeLife* align with decades of documented disparities in outcomes for Black patients, particularly those living with chronic and life-threatening conditions.

Yet this book is not written in the language of journals or policy briefs. It is written in the language of human consequence.

Yusef does something rare and powerful. He connects personal suffering to systemic failure without losing compassion, faith, or clarity. He shows us how medical trauma does not exist in isolation, but intersects with family responsibility, economic strain, geography, and history. His reflections illuminate how illness is experienced not just in the body, but in relationships, institutions, and identity.

What makes *#LemonadeLife* especially important is that it refuses to stop at survival. It insists on accountability. It challenges healthcare providers, administrators, and policymakers to confront uncomfortable truths while reminding patients and families that their voices matter—that advocacy is not optional when systems are misaligned with equity.

This book belongs in the hands of patients, caregivers, clinicians, educators, and anyone committed to a more just healthcare system. It belongs in classrooms, community discussions, and policy conversations. Most of all, it belongs wherever stories are still being dismissed as "anecdotal," despite overwhelming evidence to the contrary.

#LemonadeLife is not simply a memoir. It is testimony. It is evidence. And it is a call to do better.

I am honored to introduce this work and grateful to Yusef Harris for trusting us with his story. May it challenge us, teach us, and move us closer to the healthcare system we all deserve.

Megan Randle, DNP, FNP-C, ONS, CCRN-K, ACUE
APRN / Associate Professor / Kansas City, Kansas Community College

Introduction

The Medical Journey of Yusef Harris

There's a moment in every life when the world changes in an instant—when the life you knew slips away, and a new one begins without your permission. For me, that moment came in 2013, when I was diagnosed with Stage IV kidney failure. But the truth is, the ground had been shifting for years before that.

In 2004, my body began giving me signals—some subtle, others impossible to ignore. In 2006, a partially torn retina, which multiple surgeries couldn't repair, left me permanently blind in my left eye. It was a blow that changed the way I moved through the world, but not how I saw my purpose in it. I kept working. I kept serving my community. I kept going, even when it hurt.

When the diagnosis came nearly a decade later, it wasn't just medical—it was deeply personal. Kidney failure isn't just a physical disease. It's emotional. Spiritual. Financial. It touches every corner of your life. Dialysis became my new reality three to four days a week, tethered to a machine, sometimes feeling too sick to move, sometimes so fatigued I passed out. I lost more than energy; I lost pieces of myself. There were days I didn't want to go on—days when depression settled in like a heavy fog. Yet somehow, I kept getting back up.

Why? Because of love.

Because every time I felt like giving in, I thought of my wife, my rock, and our two brilliant daughters: both honor students, both the reason my heart beats stronger even when my body feels weak. They reminded me of the life still ahead of me. Of the power of perseverance. Of what it means to turn pain into purpose.

This book is not just about kidney disease. It's about what happens when life throws you something bitter, and you choose to make something sweeter. It's about surviving the unimaginable and somehow, finding joy. It's about choosing faith over fear and purpose over pain. This is my #Lemonadelife, not because everything is sweet, but because I've learned how to sweeten what's sour.

If you've ever faced something you didn't think you could survive, this story is for you. If you're fighting through illness, grief, or the quiet weight of being tired but trying, this story is for you.

This is not the end; this is the beginning.

When Medicine Fails the Margins

When I first received the call that a kidney was available for transplant, I thought it was the moment everything would change—the beginning of healing after years of surviving. Yet what I could not have predicted was how deeply flawed and painfully biased the system that was supposed to heal me would turn out to be.

On January 1, 2018, I underwent surgery to receive a deceased donor kidney. What followed was nearly a year of illness, confusion, and missteps by my post-transplant care team. I was diagnosed with multiple infections: E. coli, the BK virus, and CMV, though to this day, lab results have never confirmed the presence of CMV. For ten months, I was prescribed antibiotic after antibiotic, none of which were effective in treating the BK virus. All the while, one specialist—the infectious disease doctor—raised red flags, challenged decisions, and was ultimately dismissed from the team.

Then came the moment that still echoes in my memory.

I asked my nephrologist why it had taken ten months and the failure of multiple medications before they tested whether I was allergic to penicillin, an allergy I had never personally experienced or confirmed. He responded, "Because you're African American, we believed you had a stronger immune system and thought your body would fight it off on its own."

I was stunned.

"You should not be treating me based on my skin color," I replied. "You should be treating me as a human being."

What may be hardest to believe is that this wasn't just one comment. It was a window into a system where implicit bias and institutional racism are embedded in the very structure of care. The dosage of the immunosuppressant Tacrolimus—a drug known to cause kidney scarring— was never adjusted properly to account for how my body was responding. When the damage became undeniable, the truth was revealed: Tacrolimus had scarred 60 percent of my transplanted kidney. I hadn't healed. I was being harmed.

Dr. Joy DeGruy, author of *Post Traumatic Slave Syndrome: America's Legacy of Enduring Injury and Healing*, reminds us of this truth: "If you want to understand the true nature of a society, look at how it treats its most vulnerable."

In that moment and so many others, I was not seen as a patient. I was not seen as a person. I was merely a statistic, filtered through a flawed interpretation of race-based medicine. When I tried to file a formal complaint with the hospital, I was blocked, redirected, and silenced.

What I endured is not an isolated incident. It's a reflection of a medical system that still clings to outdated myths about Black bodies—myths that cost lives. It's a system that told me to wait until I returned to dialysis before I could qualify for another transplant, that disqualified me later for not meeting a weight requirement, and that never fully acknowledged the damage it had done.

This is not just my story. It is a story of many people.

#Lemonadelife is about finding sweetness in a bitter world, but it's also about telling the truth. It's about demanding humanity where it has been denied. It's about healing—not just my body, but the systems that continue to harm so many others.

This introduction begins with medical neglect, but it won't end there.

Chapter 1

The Boy Who Finished Early

Before kidney failure ever tested every ounce of my faith and fight, my life was already proof that sometimes you must learn to build something sweet out of life's bitterness, even when you're just a kid from Kansas City, Kansas, trying to make sense of two worlds at once.

I was born in July 1971 at Providence Medical Center in Wyandotte County. We lived in the Gateway Plaza housing projects off Parallel Parkway and North 5th Street. Folks around here just called it "Gateway." Those buildings were home to so many Black families trying to get by, trying to give their kids a little better than what they themselves had known.

My father landed a job at Procter & Gamble in Kansas City when I was a toddler. I'll never forget the story he tells about my maternal grandmother asking him if he was going to look for a job or lie around in her basement all day. My grandmother was responsible for taking him down to the plant to apply for a job so he could take care of my mother and me.

My mother got pregnant in college, where she met my father. They both attended Ottawa University, and by the time my mother walked across the stage to receive her college diploma, I was in her womb getting my college education as well, or so it seemed.

Quindaro

When I was about to start first grade, we moved to Brentwood. That move changed everything for me. A neighborhood with tidy yards and kids riding bikes up and down the block. That's when I started at Quindaro Elementary School, right there on North 27th Street and Farrow in the historic Quindaro Community.

It didn't take long for my teachers at Quindaro to see I wasn't like the other kids. I'd finish my worksheets before anyone else, then wander around trying to help my classmates. I got in trouble for "talking too much," but the truth was I just needed more. More to think about. More to solve.

My mother, being a teacher, was the first to challenge the system. She had to take time off work to address my constant episodes of getting in trouble in class. In reality, I would finish my work before all my classmates, and I had this urge to help them with theirs. My teachers would look up and see me at another student's desk, talking, or not at my own desk, and assume I was not doing my work or just being a troublemaker.

My mother asked the teachers about my grades. My scores were exemplary. I was getting my work done so quickly that I was bored and wanted to help others finish. My mother kindly explained that the work they were giving me was not challenging enough. So, after talking with the school principal, Mr. Leslie Brown, Sr., I was tested for the Talented and Gifted program. My test scores were stellar, so they started having me participate in a program for a select few students at Quindaro.

When they put me in the Talented and Gifted program—T.A.G., as we called it—that was my first real taste of possibility. They'd load us on buses with a small group of other kids from all over the Kansas City, Kansas Public Schools District, or KCKPS, as locals know it. They took us to a school in Fairfax with computers and foreign-language labs. I remember kids teasing me and questioning why I was getting on the short bus in the middle of the day. T.A.G. was part of the special education program, and most kids came to understand that if you rode the short bus, there was something wrong with you.

However, this education focused specifically on efficiency and creativity rather than deficiency.

From my earliest days at Quindaro Elementary to the present, I have been no stranger to disparities. From neighborhood streets to the doctor's offices, the uneven playing field of race was always there. I see it now repeating itself with my oldest daughter, who faced the same subtle and blatant inequities that once followed me. We moved our family for a better life, to build a home with my aging parents so I could help care for them. Yet even as we sought a different future, the old disparities found new ways to persist.

When my own body began to fail me, and I needed the very healthcare system that had historically neglected people who look like me, I was thrust into my own real-life education about the American medical system's racial divides.

West Middle School

By the time I hit West Middle School in the fall of 1984, desegregation was sweeping through Kansas. They shifted the system so middle school started in sixth grade instead of seventh, bringing kids from different neighborhoods and sides of town together, all learning to sit side by side.

The summer after I started middle school, I began a tailoring apprenticeship at just twelve years old after tagging along to a tailoring class with my mother. The instructor saw my interest and offered me the opportunity. While other kids played outside all day, I was learning to piece fabric together, stitch by stitch—a small introduction to the art of taking raw material and shaping it into something presentable. I got my first real paycheck, my first taste of financial freedom—money for my much-needed fashion items, including the latest tennis shoes, fabric for my own clothing creations, and the newest trendy apparel.

In middle school, I was part of the Talented and Gifted program, and it felt like everyone wanted to help me shine. I was still participating in T.A.G. at West, so I kept at it, programming, writing my first lines of BASIC code on those clunky machines. I could sketch, paint, play music, and code on a computer. There was a spark inside me that my younger years had nurtured well. It still felt like everyone wanted to help me shine.

I enrolled in art classes at West, and later, in my 7th-grade year, my art teacher—an older white woman with a keen eye—recognized something special in my pencil and brushwork. She urged my mom to enroll me in a summer program at the Nelson-Atkins Museum of Art. It was a big sacrifice for my family. My mom, a science teacher in the Kansas City, Missouri School District, would wake up early to juggle my drop-offs with the needs of my younger brother Omar and my older cousin—Harry McKelvy, who had become my adopted brother.

Harry's story was its own testament to how our family opened our doors, even when doing so made things complicated. He'd lost his twin brother to pneumonia at six months old, and then, heartbreakingly, both his parents in a car accident. After my maternal grandmother passed away, my grandfather's pastoral duties kept him on the road. The decision to adopt Harry fell to my parents, and so he became my big brother by law and by love. It brought me comfort—I was no longer the oldest. Though in truth, the weight of expectation never left my shoulders.

My mother would drop me off at the Nelson, and I remember going to my classroom and learning about different art media, styles, geographical regions, and the many painters, potters, modelers, and creative artists whose work was on display at the museum. The Nelson was an absolutely humongous property.

Every day, I had an instructional class where I sketched and learned new techniques in art media, and then we had lunch. After lunch, we would go through the gallery, observing and discussing the art and the artists. It was an entirely new style of learning that offered a hands-on, first-person look at art and creativity unlike what I was experiencing in public school.

I recognized that not everyone was getting this opportunity, and it gave me so much optimism and fed my creativity in a meaningful way. This experience immersed me in a universe I never knew existed, and while I sensed it meant something, I was taking it in with a child's understanding.

Looking back, I now realize how highly my art teacher regarded my gift at the time. My drawing skills were far more advanced than those of my classmates, and she genuinely wanted to see that talent nurtured and developed. I'm grateful my parents believed in me enough to make the sacrifices they did, and I deeply appreciate the way the people around me recognized something in me worth cultivating.

When I was about to finish up at West, my vice principal and my counselor came to our house in Brentwood, sat in our living room, and told my parents, "Yusef needs to go to Sumner Academy." Now, Sumner Academy had a reputation before it became an Academy. It was an all-Black high school when my uncle was there. After its conversion from an all-Black High School to an Academy, it became the jewel of KCK, where the district sent its brightest students to prepare them for college. They told me I'd have the best teachers, the best prep, the best shot at scholarships. Sumner went from a segregated school to an all-Black high school, then desegregated, and finally transitioned to an Academy, bringing together students from different backgrounds under one roof once again.

In 1905, Sumner became a segregated school for Black children because of an altercation ending in a white student's death. There was a segregationist sentiment in the communities of America, and this incident was a catalyst for the implementation that led to Sumner being known as an all-Black student high school.

My Uncle Darryl was a graduate of one of the last graduating classes before it became an academy. Ultimately, it became a sense of pride for the Black community and became a school known for its strong faculty and rigorous student scholastic performance. Sumner was one of the original examples of Black excellence until it was closed in 1978 as part of a federally mandated integration plan. To this day, students who attended Sumner when it was an all-Black student school hold an incredible sense of pride and self-worth regarding their attendance and graduation during those years.

However, at 14, all I knew was that my friends were going to Washington High School. I didn't want to lose them. I didn't want to have to prove myself all over again to kids I didn't know. To their credit, my parents let me decide, and I chose to stick with my friends. In hindsight, I wish I'd pushed myself and attended Sumner, but back then, it was loyalty over opportunity.

Washington High School

So, there I was at Washington High School on 7340 Leavenworth Road, home of the Wildcats—ready to see who I'd become next. There was no more T.A.G. program, but I got into more advanced math classes and computer programming. But where I really found my place was in the band room.

Mr. Ed Hoskins was our band teacher, and he was the total opposite of Mr. Wesley Lewis, the art teacher who scarred me. Mr. Hoskins was a white man who understood that the language of music was universal. He saw me, pushed me positively, and gave me every opportunity to stretch. I played in concert band, marching band, pep band, jazz band, symphonic band, orchestra—you name it. I was in it. He even let us put together a little pep band ensemble that jammed popular R&B and funk tunes at halftime of the high school basketball games.

I still remember riding those yellow buses to the KCK All-City Band events and practicing at Wyandotte High and at the old Memorial Hall near downtown KCK, the same building where James Brown and B.B. King once performed. The band room at Washington was my sanctuary when other parts of school didn't feel so safe.

Art class, though, was a whole different story. When I told my art teacher, who happened to be Black, that I wanted to apply to Parsons School of Art and Design in New York, he laughed in my face. He told me flat out, "You're not good enough to get into Parsons." I was a kid with big dreams. My dad was from Brooklyn, so I thought maybe I could live with my family and chase something bigger than KCK. That laugh stuck in my chest like a stone.

I let Mr. Wesley Lewis's words decide my future for me, and I never even applied.

I still remember years afterward when Michael Brantley called me and told me Mr. Lewis had died tragically. While you never wish for revenge by death, it seemed like a poetic ending to a time, experience, and a person in our lives that left a stain of antagonistic discouragement. We had expected him to support and understand us as young Black men, considering he was Black himself.

Music saved me. My best friend, Marqueal Jordan, who's still one of my best friends today, pulled me into the band, Harmony III. We'd practice in living rooms and basements, then perform at talent shows like the ones at Wyandotte High or the old Southeast High in KCMO. We were young musicians in a singing group on the local scene, but we had our own keyboards and drum machines. The gigs we performed at made me popular in a way that balanced out all the tough days in other classes.

High school had its share of racial and racist experiences. We were bused from 38th and Leavenworth Road all the way out to 73rd, passing F.L. Schlagle High School on our daily bus ride, even though we lived much closer to Wyandotte High on 18th Street. I was starting to experience and understand more racially motivated incidents. Washington High School was known for its iconic glass hallway, which connected two campus buildings with all-glass windows and metal framing. The glass hallway was where I experienced my first visual recognition and representation of segregation based upon color and race.

All the white students mostly mingled in the upstairs glass hallway while the Black students mingled in the lower glass hallway, where all the entertainment and culture were happening. This was 1985, and rap music was bubbling as a new musical genre, taking young Black and urban kids by storm. Hip-hop culture was taking over, and Black and Hispanic kids who had started listening to rap and watching graffiti and breakdancing in middle school were now getting up the nerve to try their creative hands at rapping, tagging, breakdancing, and creating their own offerings of the culture.

Our clothes reflected the culture: some gritty, some dressy and refined, but all making a statement about who we were becoming as teenagers. David Haskins was a premier beatboxer at the time, often serving as the rhythmic backing track for rap battles between the most up-and-coming emcees, offering their rehearsed or freestyle flows for everyone's entertainment. My neighbor and friend, John Lee, or J Lee as we called him, and Thieris Doss were two of the most polished freestyle emcees in school. Their epic daily battles provided us with something to get up to, dress up for, and look forward to in high school.

I was deeply immersed in hip-hop culture because my father was from Brooklyn, New York, and my parents sent us there for a week or two most summers. Or my Aunt Myrna and my grand-mother, Mildred Harris, affectionately known as Nanny, would send us tickets to visit. New York was an experience that got inside you and made me long for another life out on the East Coast. They made fashion, clothing, art, and music, often six months to a year ahead of the Midwest fashion trend.

I made a name for myself by bringing recorded cassettes home from New York that were copies of Friday night mixes from KISS FM and WBLS by DJs Mr. Magic and Red Alert. They were often breaking records on the airwaves and stood out from the standard radio rotation programs around the country because they were allowed to mix and scratch records "Live on Air" and remix them on the spot.

I also made a name for myself on the long bus ride to school as the warm-up beatboxer for J Lee as he entertained us with his freestyle rhymes, or I played the recorded cassette tapes I had captured while in New York for the summer with our bus driver Don's permission. Don was an older white man who allowed us to express ourselves creatively and listen to music on the bus as long as it wasn't too loud, and there was no profanity from us or the music. If we respected both him and his bus and kept it clean, he allowed us to entertain ourselves on the commute.

Every morning, we eagerly got on the bus, excited for the day's entertainment in the glass hallway. I helped J Lee and some of our later collective crew, "The Groove Boys," warm up for our daily battles.

Eric and Donnell Noel were brothers whose mom let us hang out at their house, where they had an open basement. Eric, the older brother, was a DJ and had two turntables, a mixer, and a stereo system. Eric was one of the founders of the Groove Boys and someone I looked up to. I would watch him, and he would teach me how to use the turntables. When he was done or off entertaining girls, I would get on the turntables and mix a cappella tracks with instrumentals from other records. We all rode the bus together as we learned to rap, beatbox, and entertain crowds unbeknownst to us. The bus was our breeding ground for learning how to handle ourselves in the entertainment world. It provided a safe space for us on the way to the glass hallway, where our reputations were on the line amongst our peers. Listening to the mixtapes I brought from New York was our measuring stick for how well our skills were progressing, and it let us know whether we'd be laughed at or accepted by our peers.

One day, at the steps before entering the glass hallway, I caught a glimpse of the entertainment offerings of Harmony III before I joined the group as a band member. This was where I first heard the beautiful harmonies of Harmony III and the original song "Love," which some years later seemed to be ripped off by Nelly and Kelly Rowland in their duet "Dilemma." Harmony III's current members at that time were Forrest "Dumpy" Wilson, Derek Lowe, and David Haskins, who was pulling double duty between hip-hop and R&B.

I attribute my earliest creative influences to these experiences. I wanted to, but I didn't have the confidence these talented teenagers displayed, and it took me a while to publicly beatbox in the glass hallway. I don't remember being anything but a backup when Dave or somebody else more capable wasn't around.

In gym class, I met Rodney McNeal from Oakland, California, and Marqueal Jordan from Los Angeles, California, who were both General Motors kids transplanted from the West Coast when their parents relocated to the Kansas GM plant to keep their employment tenure. As I mentioned before, Marqueal was the key to getting me an opportunity to join Harmony III, which later became Seduction

Syndicate, after Dave Haskins left Washington High and Jewel Jones joined to help fill the loss of the group's three-part harmony.

Due to the segregation of the hallway, sometimes brave Black students would try to break the barrier of the white section of the glass hallway, as we were all already participating in these integrated bus rides to school with more Caucasian and Hispanic students than we'd ever encountered in our lives. It seemed only right that, if we rode to school together on the same bus, there should be no barriers in the glass hallway. There were occasional racial attacks. Someone yelling "Nigger," or a student being antagonized for being in the wrong part of the hallway.

Over time, we built enough camaraderie that if a Black student was attacked, we all stepped in to defend them. That solidarity brought a bit of contempt among our white counterparts. I already had some exposure to white and Hispanic students in middle school. By the time I was a junior in high school, the culture had shifted to a more inclusive student body, but there were always outliers on both sides.

Rodney and Marqueal had become my best friends, but Rodney was my age, and we spent more time together. Since I was advanced in math and computing, I had quite a few classes with Marqueal's class, who was one year ahead of me. I lived in a world of broad exposure. I had a strong friendship with J Lee, who was also a year older than me, and Marqueal. Together, they introduced me to upperclassmen, with whom I built great relationships. I became well known across the student body. Rodney and I formed this bond as lower classmen, breaking through together and developing friendships with both upperclassmen and those below us.

During our sophomore year, Rodney and I saw racial atrocities and decided we'd wear black trench coats to school daily. We then wrote a manifesto regarding the protection and fair treatment of Black students and delivered it to our high school principal, Mr. Todd. In our eyes, Mr. Todd and Mr. Wren came down harder on Black students. That summer after freshman year, we played Public Enemy's *It Takes a Nation of Millions* album on repeat, fueling our activist spirits. We didn't grasp the severity of what we had done.

Mr. Butch Ellison, who I later learned was the grandson of my church's founding pastor, Naomi Haynes, was my saving grace in this moment. Mr. Ellison called me into his office, sat me down, and explained the severity of what we had done in a white world. He shared some personal stories about his days as a revolutionary. He told me he knew my parents and was sure they didn't want to discover my actions or their severity. So, he left the office, came back after talking to Mr. Todd, and that was the last time I heard of it. I learned that Mr. Ellison saw us and respected what we were fighting for, but he explained that the way we were doing things had to be rethought. He also silently informed me that he had my back. He knew I was both a good student and a fighter for equality, so we developed an incredible relationship.

There were other racial incidents during my tenure in high school. I don't need to list them all for you to understand that the world was telling me my Black body wasn't welcome but seen as a threat in certain spaces. The world was telling me I'd better watch my back.

Later, around my sophomore year or junior year, my mother purchased Polo-style shirts for my younger brother, my cousin Harry McKelvy (my adopted brother), and me. She brought them home from JCPenney's and gave them to us. None of us liked the colors she picked, so both my brothers and Rodney decided to go to the Indian Springs Mall to return the shirts for the colors we wanted, and she sent the receipt with us. We got to the mall, and since Harry was the oldest, he went to the counter with the receipt. He explained the dilemma, which the clerk acknowledged, and then exchanged the polo shirts for the colors we wanted.

When we walked out of JCPenney's after the exchange into the main hallway of Indian Springs shopping mall, we were quickly apprehended and taken to separate interrogation rooms on the lower level by off-duty police officers. They accused us of shoplifting. Each officer, after separating us, tried to get us to confess that we stole the shirts. They interrogated us and kept insisting we repeat that we had stolen the shirts. Neither of us would admit to stealing the shirts because we knew we hadn't, but we also knew that if we *had*, our parents at home were the ones we had to worry about.

Rodney, who never entered the store with us, made a life-saving decision and called our parents from the pay phone in the main halls between One Hour Photo, Italian Delight, and Topsy's. Within what seemed like minutes, I could hear my father yelling at the top of his voice, "You better let my boys out of there!" There was a lot of intense commotion, and moments later, I was reunited with my brothers as we simultaneously told my father and mother that the officers tried to get us to say we were stealing the shirts we were sent to exchange. My parents left the store with us in tow, visibly disgusted and furious. My mother attempted to contact a reputable lawyer, but nothing else came of it.

By my junior year, reality pressed down hard. I knew my parents couldn't float me through college, not with my newly adopted brother added to our household. I spent my senior year in the counselor's office, chasing scholarships. Central Missouri State University offered me a full-ride scholarship and a chance to break out, maybe land somewhere that could really see me. But a single conversation with my cousin N'Gai changed everything. He was playing basketball at Highland Community College, and the idea of going somewhere familiar—where family was nearby—felt like a safe choice. Highland offered me a partial scholarship for music after Mr. Hoskins helped me record my audition tape. The practicalities outweighed my instincts, and I signed on.

I didn't know then that playing it safe would become a habit I'd regret. Highland covered my books and tuition but left me struggling for room and board and everything else. CMSU would have given me more resources, more diversity, more opportunity, but I turned it down out of fear and the pull of comfort. I can admit now that choosing the familiar path stunted my growth. Instead of forging a new version of myself, I clung to what I knew.

The summer before my senior year, Rodney and I ran into one of the cops from the JC Penney's incident at Perkins one night while visiting our friend Tyrone Johnson, who was working there. Rodney pointed him out and let me know who he was, and though we had grand dreams of revenge, we left the restaurant without incident. We were experiencing racism in the real world now, and it didn't seem that things were going to change anytime soon.

There were a few places where my spirit found shelter—band class under the steady guidance of Mr. Ed Hoskins, and the glow of the computer lab, where coding felt like creating a new world from nothing. But the school's guidance counselors? They didn't have much of a roadmap for a kid like me. We were all just bodies to push across the graduation stage, the unique parts of us buried under paperwork and quotas.

Growing Up

Before kidney failure changed the entire trajectory of my life, my journey was already full of twists, trials, and missed turns. Looking back, my college years were not just about lectures and late nights—they were a battlefield of dreams, disappointments, and my unrelenting search for a place where I truly belonged.

By the time I reached high school, I was what folks call a jack-of-all-trades and a master of only a few. I could sketch, paint, play music, and code on a computer—there was a spark inside me that my younger years had nurtured well.

Once high school started, I was no longer the prodigy to be polished; I was just another student in the crowded halls. The same spark, carefully tended in middle school, was now left to flicker on its own. Instead of inspiring me, my high school art teacher, Mr. Lewis, made it his mission to convince me I wasn't good enough. I remember sitting in that classroom, staring at my work, hearing his voice saying I'd never make it anywhere with my talent. It cut deeper than any brushstroke could heal.

College

I graduated from high school in '89, and I had a few scholarship offers. I landed at Highland Community College up north in

Highland, Kansas, just outside Atchison. Small-town life was a shock for a city kid like me. We were so bored that we made dumb choices, like the time I got caught stealing snacks from the cafeteria.

I ran into a similar situation involving theft, and this time I was pressured to do something I knew was wrong and threatened that if I didn't participate, I would be implicated. I don't know what happened to the nineteen-year-old me. I wasn't as sure or confident about being threatened with stealing as I was when the cop told me to say I stole the shirts. I wasn't standing in the confidence that I hadn't done anything wrong, and I wasn't going to do anything wrong, despite a student of the same skin threatening me to become an accomplice in the crimes I had stumbled onto.

One of my classmates who knew me was from Detroit and played on the football team. He threatened to name me if I didn't help him, so I did. Somehow, this guy figured out that the key to his dorm unlocked the door to the cafeteria. I happened to walk in on him breaking into the cafeteria when no other students were in the adjacent activity hall.

A couple of minutes later, the custodian was walking up the hill when he saw him in the cafeteria window, even though it was supposed to be locked. The custodian saw someone else with him but didn't recognize me because he hadn't clearly seen me. I took off running and escaped the custodian's detection and apprehension. When he got caught, he gave up my name. I got expelled, lost my scholarship, and came home embarrassed and ashamed.

Back in KCK, I eventually got a job at an art framing shop called Cultural Expressions on 10th Street, right across the parking lot from Gates Barbecue. It was there that I reconnected with my good friend and classmate Michael Brantley. He'd been crushed by that same art teacher, yet he still made art his life. Michael had become an expert framer for fine art and paintings. He trained me after the owner showed me a few essential things.

We eventually felt stifled by our employers, who were a Black couple. In our opinion, they thought more highly of themselves than they should have and often kowtowed to the whims of Mr. Ollie Gates, the owner of Gates Barbecue. Mr. Gates would usually come in and chat with us, but he was only making sure we were framing his pictures correctly for his restaurant. I think he still looked at us as kids who needed supervision, but he was very nice to us, which was a little different from how our employers often treated us.

This brought Mike and me closer together as friends in the struggle of *us versus them*. I was always the meeker, less rebellious one because I was trying to live down being expelled from school for stealing, and already planning to give college another shot at the University of Kansas. I was just waiting for the spring semester to start.

Today, you'll see Mike's work at the Nelson-Atkins Museum, the American Jazz Museum, and the Zhou B. Art Center in Kansas City, Missouri, in the 18th & Vine Jazz District. Mike also runs a framing gallery called the Colour Studio, where he paints masterpieces and mats and frames paintings with an innovative, artistic flair.

When we worked at Cultural Expressions, Mike would always come up with cutting-edge matting designs that the owner frequently took credit for. The owners were African American and recognized we had talent, but it sometimes seemed to be exploited to their monetary advantage. I left Mike for college, and I was regularly his sounding board about the conditions and situations he lived through at Cultural Expressions. I always felt like I had left him all alone with no one to help bear the brunt of the adversity he faced.

Funny how the people who got knocked down with you often become the ones who stand by you longest. Marqueal and Mike, two friendships forged in setbacks, are still anchors in my life.

The University of Kansas

I was expelled from Highland in the fall of 1989 because of the theft incident. After moving back home, I worked at Cultural Expressions—a job that felt like an extension of my artistic spirit—but I knew I needed something more stable. Around that time, one of my best friends, Marqueal Jordan, transferred from Kansas State to Kansas University after a rough semester marked by relationship drama, tension with the university band director, and a classmate's suggestion that KU might offer him a better experience.

In the spring of 1990, I got a second chance, and I enrolled at The University of Kansas. I packed up for Lawrence and moved into Templin Hall with Marqueal. KU was my chance at redemption. It felt like life was saying, "You're not done yet." I enrolled at The University of Kansas with the last bit of hope that I could still pull my future together. However, KU had its own lessons in how the world could turn cold for a Black student in a predominantly white space. I joined Black Men of Today and the Black Student Union, fighting injustice on campus wherever it reared its head.

We marched when the Klan showed up. We demanded accountability when a Black female student was assaulted while delivering pizza to a Sigma Alpha Epsilon frat house. Even in my art classes, the shadows of racism crept in. I'd pour my heart into projects, only to see my white classmates get A's on work they admitted they threw together. My talent, so carefully nurtured once, was now treated as if it didn't belong.

When I moved off campus with one of my best friends, Byron Myrick from Chicago, he insisted on paying me for the first haircut I gave him, sat me down, and told me I cut hair better than any of the local barbers and that I should be charging for my craft. I had cut the Chicago skyline, or my rendition of it, in the back of his head, and word got around. Soon, our apartment became a local barbershop, and I was able to make a little money to cover food, utilities, and long-distance calls home.

He and I became local campus DJs, hired by campus fraternities and sororities to do their weekend parties. Byron knew one of the Swahili language teachers, and we'd pay him a portion of the money we made to rent his professional speakers and amps. Byron had also become the resident DJ at the college hip-hop radio station, so we got free promotional records from all the hip-hop and R&B labels, which we used to make money. I had developed some excellent mixing skills when I was part of the Groove Boys, who mostly stayed in my neighborhood when I was in high school, so by this time, that was another skill I had honed.

KU's administrative system made it worse. Twice, they left me off the academic advisors list, which meant I couldn't properly enroll in classes. The second time, desperate, I enrolled in what I thought was my next required Hausa language class (a Nigerian African language class), only to find out too late that I'd skipped a prerequisite. By the time I realized the mistake, the deadline to drop had passed. They charged me for a class I never attended.

When I finally had to leave KU in 1993, it wasn't because I failed classes; it was because I couldn't afford tuition, and I refused to go into debt with grants and loans I knew I couldn't pay back. I tried to declare myself financially independent so that my income would make me eligible for grants and scholarships. But the university treated me as a dependent of my parents and used their combined income rather than my financial circumstances.

Years later, they garnished my paycheck to cover that debt. Again, I look back on my unwillingness to go into debt for the chance to earn a degree. I realize that because of my mistakes at Highland Community College, I didn't want to burden my parents again. Out of shame, I dropped out of KU, never to enroll again.

Walking away from KU broke something in me. Highland was my chance to grow, KU was my shot at redemption, and both times I felt like I was fighting an invisible hand pushing me back down. Returning home without a degree and without my youthful confidence, I felt stripped bare. I was no longer the "special" kid; I was just Yusef, trying to make ends meet in a world that seemed determined to deny me the benefit of my own potential.

What I couldn't see then was that even in these bruising lessons, seeds of resilience were being planted. I didn't have a diploma, but I had a backbone strengthened by adversity. One day, life would test that backbone again in ways I never imagined—when my kidneys would fail and my body would betray me. Yet for now, my college story closed not with a triumphant toss of a graduation cap but with a quiet vow to keep moving forward, no matter how many times I was forced to start over.

I left KU prematurely due to a lack of funding and because I didn't want to amass significant debt. I had been given an emergency grant two semesters in a row thanks to Professor Sherwood Williams. There was a rule that an emergency grant could only be granted once, but to keep me there another semester, Dr. Sherwood Williams figured out a way to convince the school that I was worthy of two emergency grants. I spent my last semester trying to figure out how I was going to complete my degree, all the while dealing with other forms of racism.

I kept building on my love for people, helping them learn and grow. When I left school and returned home, I picked up a few odd jobs, some in sales. Feeling defeated, I decided to try to attend barber school because I had learned to cut my own hair with mirrors in high school and eventually convinced some friends to let me cut their hair. Back in college, I gave free haircuts to friends in the dorms, including student athletes.

I had developed some excellent mixing skills when I was part of the Groove Boys, who mostly stayed in my neighborhood when I was in high school, so by this time, that was another skill I had honed.

Ea La Mar's Cosmetology and Barber College

When I didn't complete a degree at KU, I headed back to Kansas City. After some research and a scholarship from Ms. Barbara McDonald at Ea La Mar's Cosmetology and Barber College, I enrolled in barber school. I went to barber school and got my barber stylist license. In barber school, I met my future wife, completed the program, and prepared to take the Missouri State Board of Barber Styling exam.

I passed the state board barber stylist exam and started looking for shops to master my craft and make a living. I graduated from barber school and started working in a suite in a beauty salon upstairs over Wings and Things on 18th and Brooklyn in Kansas City, Missouri. It was just up the street from Ea La Mar's Cosmetology and Barber College. I was still hanging out with Darrell Clark, who also attended Ea La Mar's and graduated with me.

Darrell was my transportation. We hung out together, and he dropped me off many times at the many different places I was going before and after work. Darrell eventually landed at Keith Shaw's Barbershop on 63rd and Troost and talked me into coming there to work. I still didn't have a car, so I rode the bus or asked friends for rides. I eventually moved to Missouri with another friend of mine from barber school, which made it easier to get back and forth to work.

Chapter 11

Life Before Kidney Failure

Yusef's Career, Family, and the
Onset of Health Issues

Kansas City Chiefs

My roommate would let me use his car from time to time. When he ended up on probation and house arrest, he had me drop him off at barber school and then use his car to get to work. While I was working at Keith Shaw's, I met Marc Beachem Sr., who used to cut the hair of a few Kansas City Chiefs players and would tell us about those experiences.

During this time, one of my church brothers, Albert "Alodunni" Fakeye, introduced me to Prentiss Shane, who was running N-House along with Craig Smith Sr., whose parents owned the house where the basement studio was located. I started spending my evenings in the studio, working as a producer. Michelle Lewis was a member of Onyx Pearl, a female singing group that worked and recorded at N-House Productions. I started producing and writing songs with Michelle, and we developed a great musical working relationship.

Eventually, we grew fed up with Keith Shaw's employment practices, and one of Marc's clients, Terrell Walls, offered us an opportunity to work at Hair Visions on 72nd and Troost in Kansas City, Missouri.

After working with Michelle on a few solo projects as a producer, she knew I was a barber, and one night, she called and connected me with Donnell Bennett.

Donnell explained he didn't know his way around town because he was a rookie for the Kansas City Chiefs. He was a fullback who played at the University of Miami. His current roommate, Greg, was from Texas and had played football at Texas A&M. They were both drafted by the Kansas City Chiefs in their rookie year.

After agreeing on a price for a haircut with Donnell, I decided to come to his apartment to provide my mobile barbering services.

I built a name for myself as a professional barber in Kansas City, and in my chair, I served everyone from everyday folks to Kansas City Chiefs players. I soon became the barber for many of the Kansas City Chiefs thanks to Michelle Lewis, Donnell Bennett, and Greg Hill.

When I met Greg that first night and he asked me to cut his hair, he said, "If you do a good job, you'll have a customer for life." After I was done cutting his hair, he called a couple of other players from across the hall, and that night, I made over $100 on four haircuts. Greg asked me to show up to Arrowhead Stadium the next week, and there he introduced me to Mr. Lamar Hunt and Coach Marty Schottenheimer. Kansas City Chiefs' owner Lamar Hunt and Coach Schottenheimer thanked me for taking the time to come to the stadium and keep the players looking good.

Opportunities were beginning to present themselves to me more and more. Each situation shaped my future and enriched my life experiences. The time I spent honing my talent was humbling. Cutting hair was more than just a job; it was a craft. Those moments behind the barber chair taught me about people, how to listen, how to talk, how to show up for someone even when your own life feels upside down.

Eventually, I gained Marcus Allen as a client who got a haircut weekly—sometimes even twice a week. I also started cutting Dale Carter's hair; Marc Beachem once had him as a client. Those haircuts helped me gain the business of a few veterans who had been there for a while and frequented the popular local barbershops. In time, the clientele grew and so did the perks. I often got free tickets to games in and out of Kansas City, and later I was blessed enough to meet Tamarick Vanover, whom the Chiefs had brought to the team from Canada.

Tamarick was from Tallahassee, Florida, and attended Florida State, where he repped the Seminoles and was a dynamic punt return specialist, something Kansas City hadn't seen the likes of. Every time I cut Tamarick's hair, and he ran back a kick or punt return for a touchdown, he'd tip me an extra $100 bill. He felt like my haircuts imparted a bit of good luck.

My Aunt Lillian Sumral, who lived in Wann, Oklahoma, told me that I had a cousin, Chris Penn, who played for the Kansas City Chiefs. Up until that point, I hadn't met him, but as players would frequent the barbershop where I worked, he started coming in. He was getting his hair cut by one of the other barbers, my friend and barber classmate Darrell Clark. Our barbershop had an atmosphere like the movie *Barbershop*, and our resident trash talker was the Ice Man, who we called Ice for short.

His real name was Greg Daniels. At Alcorn State, he was a baseball phenom who nearly made it to the Major Leagues but was plagued by a hamstring injury he suffered while pushing himself hard to impress a scout. He said that injury was what kept him from realizing his lifelong dream of playing professionally.

In barber school, I met a young lady who was coached by Melisa Boyd, my now sister-in-law, to entertain my advances. I wasn't the type of guy she was used to, but I was persistent with good conversation. Before long, that led to marriage and a couple of years at the Hair Visions Barber Shop. In March 1996, I married Tamika Boyd. By the fall of 1996, we were expecting a baby girl. Ultimately, I couldn't meet the demand of both places. After a misunderstanding with a Black gentleman in charge of Player Personnel for the Chiefs, I was replaced at the stadium by his local barber, DeJuan Bonds, the owner of Purple Label Barbershop and current barber for the Kansas City Chiefs and the Kansas City Royals. I felt I had no other choice but to leave the barbershop.

The reality was that barbering had its limits, so I pivoted into the corporate world. I landed at Sprint, and for a while, it felt like a second chance at the kind of success that would give my family the security I'd always dreamed of.

I didn't have any health insurance because barbers were considered high risk for coverage. Tamika didn't have good health insurance either. After talking with one of the barbershop clients, Herman Arbuthnot, I called a 1-800 number to apply for a job at Sprint, listing him as a reference. It was a sales job, something I had done before, but the benefits were too good to pass up.

Sprint

My new sales career at Sprint eventually led me into corporate training. I found purpose in standing in front of rooms full of adults, reminding them they could do more than they believed. When my daughter got older, I threw my heart into coaching girls' AAU basketball teams. I wanted those girls to hear *yes* where I'd heard *no*—to believe they were enough, even when the world told them they weren't.

My time at Sprint ended after being asked to offshore the IT help desk to Mangalore, India. I got my walking papers on December 26, 2009, the day after Christmas, ten years after I had started working there in October 1999. So many things were changing in my life. I was a new husband and father, renting a house for the first time. Then I transitioned into being a first-time homeowner. Life was constantly moving and shifting with subtle and grandiose doses of racism, which had become the permanent norm. I was a victim of predatory lending on my first home loan. Because of careful financial management and bill-paying, it never really affected my family and set the path for future opportunities.

I thrived there. I didn't just take calls; I joined the Alpha Beta team, testing systems and products before they hit the market. It brought back that Talented and Gifted feeling from my childhood—a place where people recognized my talent, curiosity, and skills.

Promotions came my way. I applied and became a corporate trainer after a conversation with one of my first corporate trainers at Sprint, Terry Loudermill. Terry made an impression on me, and I tried to figure out how to become a part of the training team. Once I became a trainer, I found one of my passions: coaching and teaching people. For once, I was shaping the work instead of just surviving it.

While my career grew, so did my family. I met Tamika while I was back in school for barbering after KU. We dated, grew together, and in March 1996, we stood before G-D and family and said, "I do." By November of that same year, we were expecting our first daughter, Naqari. In that instant, life stopped being about just me. My choices now had a ripple effect that touched my wife and the little girl we were bringing into the world.

When Naqari was born, she brought her own light. My mom, ever the educator and motivator, towed her along to community centers where she quilted. When she saw an opportunity for Naqari in basketball, she asked Tamika and me for permission to sign her up. From Saturday games at Eisenhower Middle School to my daughter towering over her classmates by sixth grade, it was clear she had a gift. By then, my parents had offered me a chance to own the house I grew up in in Brentwood, my childhood home in the Wayne Weaver subdivision. In its heyday, Brentwood was home to doctors and other professionals. Yet over the years, the sounds of the inner city crept closer: sirens, gunshots, police helicopters hovering at night. With two daughters, the urgency for a safer place grew in my chest every day. Tamika and I wanted better. She was working at a bank while my career at Sprint soared. But the demands were heavy: 6 a.m. shifts, long commutes, and the constant push to balance being good employees and even better parents. Piper School District offered open enrollment, so we leaned on my retired parents to help watch the girls. However, with my parents' retirement came a new burden: their health was slipping. My mom's diabetes had been a quiet companion for years, but now she was losing weight alarmingly fast. Sarcoidosis left her frail. My father, once a strong, sports-driven man, now struggled to catch his breath and was diagnosed with a dangerously low heart rate. I felt a duty as the oldest son, the steady bridge between my parents and my kids.

One day, while house-hunting near Piper so we could all be close, I found myself standing in a model home of a builder who had a sign on a table that read, "We'll buy your house if you buy ours." I told the builder about my plan to move into a house together with my parents to assist with their healthcare. After taking my father to look at the house and meet the builder, my father told the builder he wanted to buy a home for both of our families. My father said, "There's just one thing. My son and I both have houses to sell."

His reply? "I'll buy both your homes sight unseen." It was too good to pass up. After credit checks and walkthroughs, we realized we'd get more house for our money in Basehor, so that's where we built our dream home from scratch. In August 2007, we moved in. The girls picked out the colors for their rooms, and we watched our dreams take shape, brick by brick. It felt like a fresh chapter, a place where my kids could thrive, and my parents could find some peace.

Even so, life has a way of writing its own plot twists. By then, I had been living with diabetes since I was 23, back when I was still cutting hair. The stress at Sprint compounded things, and hypertension set in. My body was waving red flags I was too busy to notice. My primary doctor suggested I take Family Medical Leave to regroup, but it felt impossible to slow down. We were in the middle of moving, balancing new schools, new teams, and two aging parents whose needs grew as the days passed, all while raising our beautiful daughters who had their own wants and needs.

In the summer of that move, we took a family road trip from Kansas City to Chicago, then to Canton, Ohio for the NFL Hall of Fame, and finally to the Poconos in Pennsylvania to stay at my aunt Myrna and uncle Eric Williams timeshare. While playing pickup basketball with my cousins and browsing the boutiques of New York, my ankles started tingling. The swelling came and went, unexplained. I shrugged it off. A deep-tissue massage in Chicago left me in agony, but I pushed through to enjoy our family vacation.

Back home, the swelling would fade and return. My doctors had warned me that my kidneys were beginning to show signs of trouble, but I thought I could outwork it like everything else.

In 2006, I began experiencing floaters in my left eye. To take better care of my health, I went to see my optometrist, who referred me to a specialist. By October 2006, I had my first vitrectomy surgery, which left me without sight in my left eye. I went back in December for corrective surgery, but my vision still hadn't returned—though I was able to see dark shadows for about two weeks. The surgeon couldn't understand why my vision never returned. In January 2007, I had a final surgery to try to restore my vision and my eye pressure, but I lost full vision in my left eye. I continued to work at Sprint, both blind and managing lymphedema swelling.

I was later asked to research call centers in other countries where Sprint was considering offshoring the technical help desk. I ended up having to build the entire training program for agents in Mangalore, India, because my partner, who I later recommended for the corporate trainer position at the Federal Reserve, had to have gallbladder surgery.

Then came December 26, 2009. Sprint laid me off. A severance check carried us until July, and after three months of unemployment, I'd found work as a temp at the Federal Reserve Bank of Kansas City in March of 2010.

Federal Reserve

After being laid off from Sprint for three months, I was offered work. I was a corporate trainer at Sprint before coming to the Federal Reserve. I found a temp job opportunity at the Federal Reserve Bank of Kansas. I became a help desk support analyst through a temp agency placement. The agent at the temp agency was so eager to place someone in this position that she overlooked my qualifications as a corporate trainer.

After I accepted the temporary position as a help desk analyst, I was contacted by a former colleague who let me know that his recruiter was seeking leads for a corporate trainer. He gave the recruiter my name after I agreed to speak to him. The recruiter called and asked me a few questions. He assured me that he could place me in the trainer position.

I asked where it was because I had accepted the other position, as I needed to find work before my Sprint severance ran out. He told me it was at the Federal Reserve, and I told him I had just interviewed and accepted a position there. He was surprised, then said he couldn't offer me the opportunity because recruiters had a code of conduct that prohibited stepping on each other's candidates.

He asked me if I knew anyone else who was qualified, and I gave him my former co-worker's name, Kevin Leiker. I provided Kevin's contact information and then called my recruiter. I asked her why she didn't place me in the training position, but she never gave a satisfactory answer. I later found out they had a placement bonus, and things started to make sense.

After my 90-day trial run, I was denied a permanent position by my current supervisor, who was not African American but Hispanic. Every time I spoke with him about a permanent position, he would tell me it wasn't the time to convert me over to a full-time position. My wife had just started a new job at one of the many banks she worked at, so neither of us had health insurance. I kept trying to do everything I could to earn a full-time role. Yet the harder I worked and the more opportunities I took on, as my supervisor suggested, I never came any closer to the benefits package at the Federal Reserve.

One fateful day, my supervisor popped up in my cubicle and told me I needed to log off my phone. He said my wife had been in an accident, that it was on the news, and she was in the hospital. I mentioned to him that we didn't have any health insurance.

It's important to note that I had asked what I needed to do to be brought on as a full-time employee while providing excellent customer service and IT support. My manager seemed to always come up with an excuse for not recommending me for a full-time position. The very thing I was trying to avoid was happening at this very moment. He looked at me with an embarrassing look.

I drove to the hospital, upset and thinking about my wife and her well-being, but that hospital bill was front and center on my mind the whole drive there. I got there and checked on my wife, who was at Overland Park Regional Hospital. After explaining that we didn't have any health insurance and why, they finally wrote the bill off, and my wife later healed from her scrapes, cuts, and bruises.

I went back to work the next day, very upset. I later found out that my supervisor was being promoted, and I had already been on the job for more than ninety days. My supervisor called me into the office for a review before he was promoted, and he offered me a full-time opportunity for less money than I expected. I made sure to remind him of the financial medical situation since I had no medical insurance for my family.

Many other instances could have been labeled as racism at my job at the Federal Reserve, but I often took the high road and didn't call them out. I was a successful corporate trainer before working for the Federal Reserve, but they never offered me a trainer position. Instead, I recommended the person who now holds that role, and he is white.

I was required to train new analysts, but I was constantly pulled off to handle call spikes, as if I were a Super-Agent who could single-handedly take thousands of calls. After an hour or so, I was told I could resume my training classes. Those interruptions often led to longer wait times before we could fortify the floor with more trained and capable agents.

The trainer in the full-time training role had never taken any analyst calls at the Federal Reserve, but he managed onboarding, including assigning credentials and system sign-ons. When he was sick, they called me in to do his job. If I was sick, he would be incapable of doing my job, which was training analysts to take calls and support the help desk. I rarely received time off the phone to prepare for training or special projects. They expected me to perform two job titles with minimal pay and no time to prepare. When the other trainer didn't have a class, he was just in the office on the clock, getting paid to do little or nothing until the next training class.

This enforces what we're taught as Black people. You must work twice as hard to get the same pay or less to be recognized for doing the job. This theory played out in my yearly merit reviews. I was often told, "Hey, you went above and beyond on the work, but I just can't give you a 1 rating because we aren't allowed to." Sometimes I'd be compensated with a 1–3 percent pay increase for 5–10 percent more work. It became the norm.

Looking back, I was subtly conditioned to work more for less. During my tenure at Sprint, I was told my intelligence and communication style intimidated colleagues in meetings, and that I should avoid making others feel less capable.

All those years of pouring myself out for everyone else—at work, on the court, and at home—took a toll I couldn't ignore. The fatigue came first. I'd wake up more tired than when I went to bed. I remember going to work at the Federal Reserve Bank of Kansas one day. During this time, I would train a class, then be pulled out of it to take phone calls in my analyst support role.

Unfortunately, I faced further adversity as I was never allowed to hold the title of corporate trainer at the Fed. They forced me to perform tech support duties and train without the time or privilege to dedicate myself fully to that role.

Then the day came when I was so fatigued that I didn't have the strength to continue working at the Federal Reserve. I went to Human Resources, where they told me to take FMLA and see my doctor. When I went to my nephrologist, they told me the truth: I had Stage IV chronic kidney disease. I was suffering from end-stage renal disease, and my kidneys were failing.

I worked hard, just like I always did, and by September, they took me on permanently. However, my health was worsening.

My nephrologist started me on a new medication called Tekturna to help my kidneys. Instead of slowing the decline, it sped it up. Phone calls began pouring in, all telling me to stop taking the drug, as it hadn't been properly tested on diabetic patients with declining kidney function. I was living proof of what could go wrong.

By then, Naqari was busy with AAU basketball. She was on two different teams and had two practice schedules for the week. I was a

Level III support analyst by day and a corporate trainer by necessity but without the title, pay, or prep time. I was drained. One day, I sat at my desk at the Fed and quietly asked myself, *How can I keep going when my body feels like it's shutting down piece by piece?*

One day, my nephrologist called me about my labs after I had spoken to HR, and they'd advised me to take FMLA and see my doctor. January 4, 2013—I remember that date because it changed everything. I contacted him, explained my symptoms, and scheduled an appointment. I walked into the appointment on January 8, where I learned I was nearly 400 pounds and in Stage IV end-stage renal failure. I had to stop working immediately. My doctor faxed a letter to HR, and just like that, my days of powering through were over. I took FMLA and then shifted to disability. The life I'd built—the house, the family, the plans to care for my parents, the dreams of doing more, being more—had to adjust to this new reality. I was making plans to take care of my parents, but suddenly, I was the one in dire need of healthcare.

In the end, my body decided for me what my mind refused to accept: it was time to sit down. To face myself. To face my family. Learning how to live a life that would now depend on machines, on medicine, and on the unyielding hope that I could somehow make lemonade from the sourest lemons life had given me yet.

I had no choice but to walk away from the career I'd built and the people who needed me in that training room. I had to fill out the paperwork while facing the shame of the word "disability." For a man who'd spent his life giving, fixing, and building—who grew up finishing early and helping others—this was my biggest test yet: to accept help, to learn how to receive.

Yet that's the thing about a #Lemonadelife. It's not about bitterness. It's about what you do with it. Gateway, Brentwood, Quindaro, Washington High, Highland Community College, and Kansas University: all the lessons and all the losses taught me how to squeeze every drop and keep pushing forward.

And that's exactly what I'm doing now.

When I look back on my work history, I see a young man who always found a way to hustle, to learn, and to make life work even when the odds weren't in my favor. I didn't just hold jobs; I collected experiences that shaped how I navigated responsibility, family, and the quiet storms that would gather in my body long before I knew what was coming.

Yusef's Decision to Quit His Job and Go on Disability

My life up until this point had been a series of choices. Some good, some bad, but all with consequences that rippled through my family and shaped the man I was becoming. When my health began to fail, I was faced with a choice that I had never imagined I'd have to make: to give up the work I'd spent decades building and leaning on a system I barely understood.

A few days after learning I was in Stage IV end-stage renal disease, I sat in the nephrologist's office with my mother and my wife by my side, trying to process what this new reality meant. The nurse practitioner didn't sugarcoat it. She looked me dead in my eyes and told me I had three options: I could choose in-center hemodialysis, I could try home peritoneal dialysis, or I could "do nothing and die." Those words were cold, clinical, but they hit me in the chest like a freight train.

Just like that, everything I had poured into my job at the Federal Reserve, my side coaching AAU basketball, the long days balancing work and my daughters' dreams all stopped. The nephrologist had already faxed in my disability paperwork, and legally, there was no going back to work without his approval.

That wasn't coming until I had received a successful kidney transplant. Little did I know a transplant wasn't in my foreseeable future.

Still, walking away wasn't easy for me. My entire life had been pushing forward, no matter the setback. I was the child who had a hand for sketching and picking out songs from the radio with no formal training. I was the kid who'd learned tailoring at 12, the man who'd cut hair for NFL players, who'd worked and excelled at Sprint and the Federal Reserve. I created and built training programs from scratch and single-handedly researched and prepared a training program for Sprint to offshore our help desk in Mangalore, India. I knew how to forge a way out of no way.

The idea of going on disability felt like surrender. A stigma hovered over the word "disability" in my mind like I was giving up, like I was taking a handout I hadn't earned.

At my very first neighborhood association meeting at Falcon Lakes subdivision, I ran into Mr. and Mrs. Roy and Patricia Hamilton. They were family in the sense of the neighborhood, pillars of my childhood community. Mr. and Mrs. Hamilton were the parents of my younger brother Omar's good friend Adrian Hamilton and the aunt and uncle of my old friend and bandmate, Eric Davis. Eric and I spent that summer after my junior year inseparable. Hanging out, having lunch together, playing basketball, just being together as usual.

At KU, I got to know Eric's older cousin, Christopher Hamilton. Chris lived with a grace that humbled me. He was born with cerebral palsy, but I'd see him get around that massive KU campus while his roommate, Emmett Pierson, carried his books. He leaned on arm crutches, Emmett right by Chris's side to help. He never complained. At least not that I heard. We reconnected, years later, when he moved into Falcon Lakes Villas, just down the road and directly adjacent to my subdivision. We'd go to lunch, and on one of those afternoons, I opened up to him about my hesitation to file for disability due to my current health situation. I didn't want to lose income, but even more than that, I dreaded the label.

Chris listened. Then he told me what his mother, Mrs. Hamilton, told him to share with me, gently but firmly: the money wasn't charity, it was insurance I'd paid into my whole working life. He told me I should be proud to qualify, not ashamed. Then he leaned in closer and said something I'll never forget: "Yusef, you lived your whole adult life standing tall. I was born with my disability, but you? You built a life, a family, a career. Now you're fighting a new battle you never asked for. Don't be ashamed to get the help you deserve."

Mrs. Hamilton's words through Chris reminded me that disability was part of the safety net I'd earned and wasn't a handout, but a lifeline. I sat across from Chris at that table, his words echoing inside me. I felt the tears before I realized they were falling, rolling down my face, hot and slow. Sometimes pride is the heaviest thing a man can carry. That day, Chris and Mrs. Hamilton helped me put mine down.

So, I signed the paperwork. The Federal Reserve processed my short-term disability while the Social Security Administration reviewed my case for permanent long-term disability (LTD). I went from steady paychecks to 40 percent of my salary, a number that stung even worse because I'd spent years hearing excuses about why my dedication never translated into a pay scale that reflected my work. I never earned a raise other than "cost of living," nor did I receive a salary raise or merit raise from my personal contributions, skills, and sacrifice. But numbers didn't matter anymore. Survival did.

That day, I returned to the nephrologist for my education appointment. My mother and wife sat beside me as the reality of dialysis settled in. I would need a fistula, a direct connection between an artery and a vein in my left arm, my non-dominant side. It was my gateway to staying alive. The first fistula failed to mature properly, so I needed a revision and a graft added.

On April 13, 2013, I had my first dialysis treatment in the hospital, and a caseworker set me up for in-center dialysis. That day marked the death of the life as I had known it. I had to give up the job that once made me feel seen, the coworkers who felt like family, the possibility of promotions, and the hustle of early mornings in the office. I had to let go of coaching my daughter's basketball teams, the thrill of watching her outgrow her rivals on the court, and the simple joy of the everyday life I'd grown accustomed to. Dialysis became the new center of gravity around which my life and the lives of the three women I loved most—Tamika, Naqari, and Miyala—now orbited.

Walking away from my career and stepping into this new life felt like standing at the edge of a cliff I hadn't asked to climb. Though deep down, I knew I didn't climb it alone. The community that raised me, the lessons from my parents, my kids, my wife, my church family, and the gentle words of a friend born into a battle he never chose—they all pushed me to see that my worth was never just my paycheck or job title. It was in my resilience, my love, and my refusal to let kidney failure have the last word.

So, with all the fear and uncertainty, I stepped onto this new road—fistula scars in my arm, disability checks in the bank, and the fragile hope that even now, I could find a way to make lemonade out of the lemons life kept throwing at me.

Chapter 111

The Harris Dilemma

The Special, Prepared Ladies

The Girls

I spent much of my twenties carrying a quiet resentment—toward choices I'd made, toward circumstances I couldn't control, and if I'm honest, toward my parents too. I was grateful for the stability and the sacrifices they made for us, but in the stubborn corners of my young mind, I thought about long mental lists of everything I would do differently when it was my turn to be a father.

What I didn't understand back then was that parenting isn't a job you arrive perfectly prepared for. You learn as you go. Even by the time you've raised a second, third, or fourth child, you're still stumbling your way through, adjusting, patching up mistakes with love and hope that you'll get it right the next day. Only later, when you become a grandparent—if you're lucky enough to live that long—do you look back with gentler eyes, recognizing all the small ways you did your best and all the ways you wish you could have done more.

I didn't know then that this stubborn, critical way of thinking would become the very thing that shaped me into the kind of father I wanted to be—present, protective, and always striving to do better for my girls.

Growing up, there were parts of my childhood that gave me permission to dream. Being in the Talented and Gifted program was my first taste of that freedom. T.A.G. let me imagine a life without fences, a world where I could be whoever I wanted. Even so, each afternoon, I'd step off that little bus and back into the real world. A world of limits, rules, and the unspoken reminder that a gifted Black boy from the Projects shouldn't expect too much.

At home, no one made a fuss over me being "special." They couldn't. My parents had three sons to raise, each of us carrying our own needs and burdens. In our house, love was equal parts survival and fairness. Yet, even as we left the Projects and settled into the suburbs, something inside me stayed restless, driven by the same spirit that would one day lead me door-to-door asking neighbors if they needed their grass cut, their snow shoveled, or their leaves raked for a few dollars to pocket for my own desires.

That spirit of working, hoping, and pushing forward became a seed I would pass down to my daughters, whether or not they asked for it. I didn't truly understand how my own struggles would touch my children until my first daughter, Naqari, arrived. The selfishness that had colored so much of my young manhood left me the moment she took her first breath. She was a bright-eyed baby girl, born with steel-gray eyes that would shift like the seasons—sometimes hazel, sometimes green. Every now and then, a glint of that same gray would peek through, reminding me how special she truly was.

Naqari, My Firstborn

Naqari came into this world with a veil over her face, a rare sign in our family, though I didn't know it at the time. As I watched the doctor lift that delicate membrane away, I had no idea it was meant to be saved, dried, and pressed into a Bible—a sacred token of the child's gift to see beyond what the rest of us can. When I told my mother about it afterward, she emphatically asked, "Where is it?"

I explained that the doctor had discarded it after he lifted it from her face. She looked so disappointed. "That veil," she said. "You were supposed to keep it. Children born with a veil can see things others can't!"

At first, it felt like a strange old wives' tale—something whispered through generations. However, when Naqari was about four, I learned just how real it was. We were driving our usual route to church, taking Highway 71 South to 39th Street in Kansas City, Missouri, when she started pointing at nothing and saying, "Mommy, the baby girl," dragging her tiny thumb across her throat. We didn't understand. She did it repeatedly, each time with wide, worried eyes that seemed far too old for her little body.

It wasn't until years later that the story of Erica Michelle Marie Green—known to the world as Precious Doe—unfolded. We realized what our baby had been trying to tell us. For whatever reason, when we passed through that corridor, she was compelled to tell us about a baby girl who had been murdered unbeknownst to us. The truth of that tradition, that gift, revealed itself in that heartbreak. Over the years, Naqari would have other visions, some she shared, many she kept close to her heart. It was a heavy gift for a gentle soul. Yet she has always carried it with quiet grace and a deep love for the world around her.

Miyala, My Baby Girl Princess

Then came Miyala—my Baby Girl Princess. She was born five years after her sister, in the fall of 2001, a soft and knowing soul from her very first breath. Where Naqari's gift felt like an ancient spirit that hovered at the edge of the unseen, Miyala's gift was her intuition, her gentle wisdom that seemed far beyond her years.

When she was only three, she could explain the meaning of the word "prototype" to her grandfather after hearing "Prototype" by Andre 3000 so often on the radio and music video stations. It seemed like such a small moment, but it revealed something big: her mind was always reaching, always grasping for the bigger picture.

When life knocked me down, Miyala's love lifted me up. I remember one of my darkest moments recovering from the surgeries that stole the vision in my left eye. The pain was so fierce it drove me to my knees. There on the floor, on my knees at the back of a Walgreens pharmacy, tears blinded what little sight I had left. I was in so much pain that I asked the pharmacist to give me one dose of the medication he was filling. I was denied. I was literally on my knees, blood seeping through the bandage covering my eye, crying. And there she was. My little girl, tiny hands rubbing my back, her soft voice breaking through my sobs: "God, please help my daddy. God, please help my daddy."

Her love poured over me like medicine no doctor could ever prescribe. She has always been my quiet reminder that even in my brokenness, I am seen. I am loved. I am needed.

The pain continued even after I got home from the pharmacy. When we got into the house, Miyala went to her bedside, unprompted and unassisted, dropped to her knees, and started praying so sincerely and earnestly on behalf of her daddy. The prayer was so intense and intentional that I knew G-D could not resist her petition and that I would be okay.

My daughters are my special, prepared ladies. Bright, perceptive, and strong in ways I could never have imagined. They are proof that even when life tries to take everything from you, it cannot steal the love that binds a father to his girls, nor the gifts they carry forward. Gifts they were born with, gifts they carry for us all.

My Sunshine Tamika

When I speak about the special women who've held me up through life's hardest seasons, I would be remiss if I didn't tell you about Tamika Harris—my wife, my Sunshine, my anchor when the storms rolled in.

What many people see today is a devoted, nurturing woman, but what they don't always know is that before she ever carried my burdens, she had already survived storms of her own. When Tamika was just a teenager, the youngest of six children, her world was turned upside down. Her father, Herman Boyd Sr., had to undergo a heart transplant during her senior year of high school. While her older siblings were grown and out on their own, Tamika was at home, the last one left, holding down the fort with her mother.

She should have been out dreaming big dreams, picking out colleges, giggling with her girlfriends about prom dresses and senior year crushes. Instead, she sat beside her father's hospital bed, helping him fight for each new heartbeat, each small step toward recovery. After enrolling in community college, when her mother needed her most, Tamika made the heartbreaking decision to drop out in her first semester and get a job to help support the household. She sacrificed her own plans to care for the man who'd always spoiled her, protected her, and loved her like only a true daddy's girl could understand.

When her father passed away, it left a wound in Tamika that never truly healed. I didn't know any of this when we first met. Back then, I only knew she carried a quiet strength behind her warm, broken smile—a standard of love and loyalty that would set the bar for every man who hoped to love her.

I learned about heartbreak years later. During Tamika's season of mourning, she discovered her first love was not the man she thought he was. Already crushed by the loss of her father, she pulled into a gas station one day, a routine stop for gas and maybe a bag of chips, only to find her boyfriend's truck parked out front, another girl sitting in the passenger seat. It was the kind of moment that makes you question everything you thought you knew about love and trust.

Yet when I met her at Ea La Mar's Cosmetology and Barber College, I never saw that brokenness. I just saw a woman who carried herself with grace, a quiet resilience wrapped around her like a second skin. I was the kid who'd always run headfirst into challenges, so when I set my sights on her, I made up my mind that I'd earn her love, even if it took every ounce of my persistence.

Melisa, my sister-in-love, likes to remind me that I owe our marriage to her. She was my biggest champion, always campaigning on my behalf, whispering in Tamika's ear to give me a chance.

Tamika still reminds me that she had no interest in me at first, and Melisa still takes credit for changing her mind. After many sentimental cards, love letters, and other advances, she finally gave in.

Though winning her heart was only the beginning, what Tamika has given me since then is beyond anything I could have imagined. She was my caretaker when I was too stubborn to care for myself. She was the steady force behind every doctor's visit I didn't want to make, every medical bill I didn't think we could afford, every moment I needed a push to put my health first.

She showed that same devotion when she drove me to work and back every single day for months after I lost vision in my left eye. It sounds simple. What's a ride to work between a husband and wife? But that ride wasn't down the street. It was a daily testament to her sacrifice. She'd drive me all the way to South Kansas City, Missouri, then drive back to 7th and Minnesota Avenue to work her full-time job in Kansas City, Kansas. After her shift, she'd make the same long trip again to pick me up and take us back to the home we paid a mortgage on in Kansas City, Kansas. She did that every morning and every evening for months until I learned to drive with one good eye. On top of that, she did it without complaint, without ever making me feel like a burden, even as she shouldered her own work and our family at the same time.

Long before that, when she was pregnant with our first daughter, Naqari, Tamika faced her own brush with fear. I still remember the gut punch I felt when I learned she had fainted at her teller station at the bank—passed out cold from undiagnosed gestational diabetes. We didn't have cell phones then, just pagers, and it took a while before someone got the message to me that there was trouble. I couldn't protect her that day, just like I couldn't protect her when that same bank where she worked so hard was robbed. She stood at her counter, forced to smile through her fear, while a man with a gun demanded her cash drawer.

The man passed a note to her that read, "Give me the money in your drawer. Large bills only, no
$20s. I have a gun. Be quiet and don't reach for the button. Pass the note back when you're done." The man kept a jovial smile on

his face the entire time as he was robbing the bank and her. After he left, she notified her coworker that she had been robbed. She didn't believe her at first, but when everyone realized the bank had been robbed, they called the police. Tamika called me and told me what happened. So, I left work immediately and picked her up. She was visibly shaken. I did my best to console her, but this was the second time I couldn't be there to protect her.

Each time life threatened to shatter her spirit, Tamika stood up straighter, prayed harder, and somehow kept on giving her love away like a gift she would never run out of.

Even in the smallest moments, she showed her devotion. After that scare at the bank, we went out together and got our first cell phones. It might seem trivial now, but back then, picking our own phone numbers that ended in the same four digits as our home address felt like a promise

that no matter what, we would always be reachable for each other and for the children we would raise together.

Tamika is more than a wife to me. She is proof that love isn't just sweet words and romantic gestures. Real love is a quiet ride to work when you can't see straight. It's sitting at a hospital bedside when you should be planning your own future. It's standing at a teller counter with a gun pointed at you and going home to love your family anyway.

In every moment life has tried to knock us down, Tamika has been my light, my comfort, my Sunshine. The kind of woman who makes you believe that no matter how bitter life gets, there will always be someone who knows how to turn lemons into lemonade.

Yusef's Experiences with Dialysis and the Toll on His Family

Dialysis was supposed to keep me alive, but every session reminded me just how fragile life could be when your own body betrays you.

In the beginning, I didn't know how hard it would hit me. Within the first few weeks, I found myself coming in and out of consciousness, my blood pressure dropping so low that the nurses had to elevate my feet above my head to keep me from slipping away. One moment I'd be sitting there staring at the television, trying to distract myself; the next, I'd wake up confused, looking at the ceiling while people hovered over me, trying to bring me back.

Then there were the cramps. The kind of pain that doesn't just throb, but grabs hold and wrings you out until you're ready to scream. It started in my legs, an ache from being stuck in that recliner for four long hours, unable to stretch or move enough to be comfortable. The worst came when the stomach cramps hit. It felt like invisible hands were digging into my gut, twisting my muscles like a wet rag. I'd shoot up from my chair, desperate to stand tall, trying to stretch out the agony, but there was no real relief. Although it was the natural reaction to stand up and seek comfort, it was dangerous to rise so suddenly, as blood rushed back into circulation after hours of stagnant reclining or sitting.

It wasn't just the treatments themselves. Dialysis seeps into every corner of your daily life. Every sip of water becomes a calculated risk. I was supposed to limit myself to 32 ounces of fluid a day—not just water, but every ounce of soup, every bite of fruit. Some days I'd sit at a restaurant with a glass full of ice, waiting for it to melt so I could trick myself into thinking I was quenching my thirst. You never know real thirst until you must measure every drop.

And right when you think you're settling into a routine, the chairs start emptying. One by one, the people you see every week— the men and women who become your brothers and sisters in the dialysis fight—sometimes don't show up for treatment. Some slip away quietly. Others, like one patient I'll never forget named Michael, come in to say goodbye when they know it's their last treatment. I watched that man say goodbye to everyone in the room because the calcification of his organs meant there'd be no coming back tomorrow. It was gut-wrenching. Dialysis doesn't just break down your body; it chips away at your spirit every time you do it and every time someone's chair is empty.

Some days, I didn't make it to dialysis at all because I was in the ER with pneumonia again. My failing kidneys couldn't flush the extra fluid, so it filled my lungs instead. Those were the weeks I had to get daily dialysis in the hospital, fighting to breathe while still tethered to that machine.

Then there were the trips to the access center. I'd lie on a cold table, half-sedated as they inserted an IV line to balloon open the narrowing in my fistula or to place stents into my arm. My body was always trying to heal itself, closing the fistula that was supposed to keep me alive. If the fistula clotted or narrowed, the treatment didn't work. No treatment meant more fluid buildup, more hospital stays, and more setbacks that kept me off the transplant list.

Dialysis demanded everything. I was always pushing toward my dry weight goal, trying to prove to the doctors that my body could handle a new kidney. At the same time, I was trying to be a father—figuring out how to travel for out-of-town AAU basketball tournaments so I could support my daughter, even when I was too weak to stand for long.

I'd look in the mirror and barely recognize myself. My skin darkened. My eyes turned hollow and weary. I got into car accidents because I was so exhausted that my brain lagged behind my reflexes. Dialysis was sucking the life out of me—literally.

By 2016, two years in, it hit me like a Mack truck. My blood pressure was sky-high, my legs swollen and disfigured, my hope wearing thin. Still, I refused to give up. I fought back with every ounce of energy dialysis hadn't stolen yet. I started walking on the treadmill—fifteen minutes at first, then thirty. I walked laps in the pool, then did water aerobics. On non-dialysis days, I hit the YMCA to lift weights and do cardio, fighting through the fog in my head and the ache in my bones.

Every step was a desperate prayer: *Lord, let this get me closer to my transplant.* Dialysis was the price I paid to stay alive long enough to get that second chance. Yet every session, every cramp, every hospital stay reminded me that the fight for survival takes so much more than just showing up. It takes every drop of your will to keep living, even when life is draining out of you, one treatment at a time.

If you want to truly understand how chronic illness weaves its fingers through every corner of a family, you need to look at what dialysis did to mine—not just to my body, but to the hearts and hopes of the people who loved me most.

My youngest, Miyala, was only a little girl when she had to watch me shrink into someone who was often too weak to even stand up straight. She has told me it broke her spirit to see the toll dialysis took on me, how it made me sick and worn and gray around the edges. She was just a child trying to live her own life, yet every trip I made to that cold chair in the dialysis clinic made her worry whether I'd ever get a new kidney or if I'd be stuck in that cycle forever.

She carried fears no child should bear: Would her Daddy make it back home each day after driving himself to and from those treatments? Would he be too tired to pick up her big sister, Naqari, who had her own battles to fight at an age when she should have been carefree?

It still stings to say it, but dialysis didn't just rob me of my energy—it robbed my oldest daughter too. Naqari's freshman year at Basehor-Linwood High School was supposed to be a time for her to shine on the basketball court and in the classroom. Instead, she faced hate in its ugliest form in addition to learning to navigate with a father on dialysis.

It started when she left her homework folder in class one day. When she got it back, it had a crude drawing of a penis and a swastika scribbled inside. She brought it home to us, looking for protection. I felt helpless. I'd moved my family to that school district, believing its high test scores meant better opportunities for my kids. I didn't know I was leading her into a nightmare.

When Trayvon Martin was murdered, the wound of living while Black felt raw for all of us, but it was a constant fear for me. As I drove Naqari to school and then to two different AAU basketball practices, every radio talk show we listened to replayed Trayvon's story on a loop: a Black child, gunned down for wearing a hoodie and daring to exist in a neighborhood where he "didn't belong." I looked at my own daughter—brilliant, driven, talented—and wondered if I would ever be enough to keep her safe.

I tried. I called the Basehor police to my home with evidence in hand. They explained they couldn't handle incidents that happened on school grounds. They told me to have her report it to the school resource officer. She did, and nothing happened. Then, a boy in the cafeteria walked past her and yelled out the word that cuts deeper than a blade: "Nigger!" Many students laughed. Teachers shrugged it off. Even the teammates I'd coached—girls I'd spent time, money, and heart on—stayed silent. I couldn't believe my daughter was alone at that moment.

When someone vandalized her decorated basketball locker with profanity, that was the final blow. Three incidents, three times my child came home hurt. Three times I had to swallow the rage that comes when you can't protect the people you love most.

We transferred Naqari out of Basehor and into Leavenworth High School, a more diverse community in a military town, though even that decision turned into a fight. The same people who had ignored our calls and denied racism even existed in their school suddenly wanted to stop her from leaving. They filed an injunction claiming she'd been "recruited" for basketball. I was livid. I wasn't fighting for trophies. I was fighting for my daughter's sense of self, her right to feel safe just walking down the hallway.

In the end, they couldn't stop her. My daughter turned her pain into fuel. She made Leavenworth High proud. Three state championship basketball finals, back-to-back Kansas 6A State Championship rings, and a scholarship named in her honor at Leavenworth High School. She went on to play basketball at Coffeyville Community College, then earned her bachelor's degree in social work from KU, where she was chosen to give a graduation speech that left me in tears of pride. Yet underneath all her success, she still carried the memory of driving home with me after dialysis sessions, watching me struggle to stay awake behind the wheel. She says now that it hurt her soul to know how much I was suffering, even while I was trying so hard to hold up the rest of the family.

Tamika—my Sunshine—saw it all. She was tired too. Tired of the hospital stays. Tired of watching my body fail me. Tired of the way dialysis would flood me with fluids one day and drain me dry the next. So many nights she stayed up late, wrapping my swollen legs in layers of foam and bandages because my lymphedema had grown so bad my legs doubled in size. Every morning, she'd get up early to do it all over again.

When she looked at me on that dialysis bed, it brought back all her old scars. Memories of her father hooked up to machines after his heart transplant. Memories of the sacrifices she made, the dreams she left behind to take care of someone she loved. Now, here she was again, watching me fight for every drop of energy.

I wasn't the only one hooked up to that dialysis machine. My wife and my daughters were all tethered to it too. They each paid for it in their own way: in tears shed in the dark, in sacrifices made without question, in the quiet strength it takes to keep loving someone who might not be here tomorrow.

If you want to understand what chronic illness costs a family, don't look at the needles in my arm or the swelling in my legs. Look at the tired eyes of my wife. Look at the worry etched into my daughters' faces. Look at the sacrifices they made to keep this family together when I couldn't.

This is the truth of our #Lemonadelife: Sometimes the people who hold you up are the ones who carry the heaviest weight. And yet, somehow, they never let it break them.

Unveiling the Disparities in Healthcare Access and Treatment

Writing and Documentation

The following documentation illustrates some of the most atrocious historical examples of disparities, racism, and racial bias in modern medicine. Some examples illustrate how Black bodies—men, women, and children—were robbed of their humanity, dehumanized, and animalized. It's horrifying to realize the mental disassociation and madness that had to be rationalized to justify the horrors that advanced modern medicine at the expense of Black lives!

Yusef's Personal Discoveries

From my earliest days at Quindaro Elementary to the present, I have been no stranger to disparities. From neighborhood streets to the doctor's offices, the uneven playing field of race was always there. I see it now repeating itself with my oldest daughter, who faced the same subtle and blatant inequities that once followed me. We moved our family for a better life, to build a home with my aging parents so I could help care for them. Yet even as we sought a different future, the old disparities found new ways to persist.

When my own body began to fail me, and I needed the very healthcare system that had historically neglected people who look like me, I was thrust into my own real-life education about the American medical system's racial divides.

The Allergy That Wasn't

One of my earliest personal discoveries happened during my first kidney transplant journey. When I was a child, my mother was told I was allergic to penicillin. Like many Black families then, we did not question the doctors. We took what they said as gospel. From then on, whenever a nurse or doctor asked about allergies, I faithfully told them, "I'm allergic to penicillin."

Fast forward to my kidney transplant: I got E. coli, was misdiagnosed with CMV, and had abnormal BK virus numbers. The medical team scrambled for treatment options, yet with penicillin off the table, they struggled for nearly a year to find alternatives, while my new kidney and I suffered. It wasn't until my post-transplant nephrologist finally asked me, "What happens when you take penicillin?" that the truth started to unravel.

I realized no one—not even I—actually knew. My mother had been told that when I was a baby. Ten months, three kidney biopsies, two hospitalizations, endless antibiotic trials, and a new infectious disease doctor later, I was finally sent to an allergy specialist.

They injected penicillin under my skin. I waited. No reaction. Then they prescribed me amoxicillin and told me to take it immediately. Again, nothing. After a lifetime of believing I carried a dangerous allergy, I discovered I wasn't allergic at all. This was one of the most anxiety-ridden tests I had ever experienced. I had no idea what penicillin did to my body, but I suspected it could be dangerous, even life-threatening. For the first time in my entire life, I would find out what penicillin did to me.

It was a lesson in how an unchecked note in a chart can cascade into years of misdiagnoses, unnecessary suffering, and delayed care, and how assumptions about Black patients' resilience or biology can shape decisions without our input.

From Anxiety to Advocacy

Those ten months were some of the hardest of my life. I was overwhelmed by a maze of specialists, contradictory opinions, and failed treatments. A nurse, seeing me falling apart and overwhelmed, suggested I talk to someone about how I felt. I took her advice, though at first my therapy experience fell short. Each week, my therapist—a white woman—listened but offered no tools, no context for my feelings of despair and anxiety. She would repeatedly say in each session, "You sound like you have a good handle on things." But I didn't. I was drowning.

Years later, I found my true therapist—an African American man from my community. He knew my world and spoke my language. He explained what happens in the brain and body when you experience anxiety. He presented me with tools to manage my anxiety and showed me the difference real cultural understanding makes in mental healthcare. He told me to write about what happened to me and explained that it would help me heal and maybe help someone else avoid what I endured.

Patterns That Repeat

Through all of this, I noticed a pattern: doctors often assumed I wouldn't do the work to get better. Many seemed invested in treating my symptoms, not helping me break free from the cycle of disease. I once asked an endocrinologist to refer me to a dietitian. He shrugged. "You don't need one." That was my very last appointment with him. I knew then that finding the right providers meant finding people who would see me as a partner, not a stereotype.

Still, the old ideas persisted. When I finally asked my post-transplant nephrologist why they had waited ten months to send me to an allergist, he said, "Studies show African Americans have stronger, almost superhuman immune systems. We were waiting for your immune system to kick in and handle the viruses."

My father was sitting right next to me when I fired back, "Don't treat me based on the color of my skin. Treat me like a human being."

That moment marked the start of my deep commitment to advocating for myself and others who look like me. After ten months of missteps, the real culprit turned out to be Tacrolimus, a drug that suppressed my immune system to the point that my new kidney never recovered. By October, my new kidney was 60 percent scarred. There was no coming back. Today, I'm required to visit an outpatient infusion center every 28 days, receiving a Belatacept drip through a vein in my arm to prevent my kidney from being rejected. I've learned to push for answers, push back when needed, and be my own loudest voice in every room.

Generational Burdens, Generational Healing

If my life has taught me anything, it's that the injustices of the past—Sara Baartman, the Tuskegee Experiment, Henrietta Lacks, eGFR bias—are not just distant history. They echo through every misdiagnosis, every dismissive provider, and every moment when a Black patient must fight twice as hard to be heard.

Yet by telling my story—by writing *#Lemonadelife*, the book—I hope to show that the legacy of exploitation and neglect doesn't have to be our future. My hope is that my journey helps others find their voice, stand up for their care, and never again accept being treated as less than human.

Connecting the Dots

This is how my personal discoveries connect with the writings and documentation of healthcare disparities. They are not separate chapters. They are the same story, unfolding across centuries—a story that must be told, so that we might finally write a different ending.

Together, these documented histories and modern cases show how deeply systemic racism is woven into healthcare. From Sara Baartman's dehumanization to the exploitation of enslaved women by medical pioneers, the theft of Henrietta Lacks' cells, the Tuskegee deception, to algorithmic bias in kidney transplant eligibility. Each story reveals how institutions have used Black bodies as resources while denying them equitable care.

Chapter IV

#Lemonadelife Day

The Day of Unexpected Circumstances

January 8, 2013—that date is tattooed in my memory. It was the day I heard the words that turned my world upside down: Stage IV end-stage renal disease. I remember sitting there, feeling like the walls were closing in, my mind racing through every responsibility I carried on my shoulders. My kidneys were failing. My kidney function had plummeted to just 15 percent. I had to stop working immediately.

I'd built a life I was proud of. A full-time corporate trainer and Level III IT Support Technician, juggling complex demands and problem-solving all day, every day. Providing for my family had always been my promise, my pride. Now that stability felt like it was crumbling under my feet.

At home, my daughters were charting their own journeys. My oldest, Naqari, had just wrapped up her time at Coffeyville Community College, where she played basketball and made us so proud. She chose not to continue the sport at KU, instead pouring all her energy into her academic and Social Work major. Miyala, my youngest, was finding her footing at

Basehor-Linwood High School. She decided she wanted to continue with her classmates, and we allowed her to, but we did so with an unspoken pact: if racism or bullying touched her, we'd pull her out in a heartbeat. No question. I did so with trepidation, wonder-

51

ing how much of a difference five years would make. I had spent my whole life facing the reality of racism; I would not allow my baby girl to carry that burden alone.

Meanwhile, dialysis became my new full-time job. One that didn't pay, didn't care, and didn't get easier: Monday, Wednesday, Friday. Each treatment left me exhausted, my body fighting to feel normal again. They told me when I started that dialysis was like running a marathon without physical activity. They weren't lying. It felt like my heart and my hope were being drained one cup of blood at a time, only to be fed back in again, as if my life was on a slow, constant drip cycle.

On my off-days—Tuesday, Thursday, Saturday—I fought to keep my body and mind from sinking. I built myself a creative and entertainment haven in the basement of our home after we moved to Basehor—my man cave. It was my sanctuary, my escape. There was a music studio to record my thoughts and musical creations, a little barbershop corner to keep my skills alive, and my pride and joy—a movie theater setup with a 100-inch screen and surround sound that helped me escape and forget, if only for a while. I'd spend my mornings on the treadmill for thirty minutes, head to the neighborhood pool for laps, then finish the day with another walk on that treadmill. Each routine gave me something to look forward to, a reason to get up.

Ironically, even my sanctuary had its flaws. The basement was concrete on all sides, built like a bunker. The one thing it couldn't hold was a cell phone signal. No matter how hard I tried, calls would drop, voices would fade to static, and every important conversation I attempted down there would end in frustration. Over time, I stopped expecting my phone to work in that space. It was just another limitation I had to accept.

That bitter acceptance grew over nearly five years of waiting for a kidney that never seemed to come. Being on the transplant list meant I always had to stay within four hours of my transplant hospital. My freedom shrank to a tight circle on a map. Traveling to see Naqari play basketball during her high school years required strategic planning. Later, traveling to Coffeyville, Kansas, to see her play basketball became another planning session, given that the college was three and a half hours away. Finding dialysis centers wherever we went, submitting paperwork, taking tuberculosis skin tests, and arranging every detail so I could stick to my schedule. There was no such thing as a spontaneous family trip. Every mile I traveled carried the fear of missing that one life-changing phone call.

So, when December 2017 rolled around, and I was still tied to the dialysis chair, a piece of me quietly laid that hope to rest. We'd made it our tradition to go to Watch Meeting on New Year's Eve—a service where we gathered at church, gave thanks for the year's blessings and burdens, and prayed in the new year with songs and hope for better days. But that year, a harsh ice storm canceled the service, leaving us to pray on our knees at home instead on New Year's Eve.

I remember that day so clearly. Naqari called from KU to say she wanted to come home on New Year's Day. I told her firmly not to. The roads were slick with ice and very dangerous. She was alone. I trusted that she'd listen. She always did.

That night, around 7:45 p.m., I headed down to my basement haven with my phone in hand, knowing it was basically dead weight down there. I turned on the projector, powered up the surround sound theatre system, and settled onto the futon behind the coffee table, ready to drown out my thoughts with a good movie. My wife and Miyala were planning to join me once everything was set up. I laid my phone on the coffee table, not even giving it a second thought.

Then, suddenly, in that concrete tomb where calls never survived, my phone rang. It rang!

I picked it up almost on reflex. "Hello?" I said, expecting static or silence. Instead, a clear, calm voice answered back. She was calling from St. Luke's Transplant Center. I was number two on the list. There was a deceased donor with two viable kidneys. If I was willing, I needed to get to the hospital by 9 p.m. sharp.

I sat there, frozen for a second. Five years of waiting, praying, planning my life around a maybe, and here it was. I walked out to the downstairs living room, still calm, and told my wife and daughter the news. At first, they thought I was joking. I've played plenty of pranks over the years. They thought maybe this was another. But when I told them to grab my emergency bag, their eyes widened. The reality sank in.

Right then, the front door creaked open. I heard a familiar voice. My stubborn, fearless Naqari, a key rattling in the lock as someone was letting themselves in. "Naqari, is that you?" I yelled up the stairs.

"Yes, Dad," she called back, like it was nothing, but it was everything. I'd told her not to come home. Despite that, she showed up anyway. Now she was here to accompany her father to the hospital for a transplant that would hopefully give him back the life that kidney failure had tried to steal. To this day, I wonder if she had some intuition that motivated her to defy my orders. How does this veil work exactly?

My father, who hardly ever went down to the basement because of his hip replacements, came down the stairs, hearing the commotion. I went halfway up the stairs to tell him the news. He followed me downstairs in disbelief, asking over and over, "Are you serious, man?"

My girls and my wife—all of us moving, packing, heading to the hospital. I slipped on my #Lemonadelife T-shirt, the one that reminded me every day that when life hands you lemons, you squeeze every drop and make something sweet.

It wasn't just a saying; it was my armor. As we traveled from Basehor, Kansas, to the St. Luke's Plaza location in Kansas City, Missouri, I instructed my wife and daughter to call people I knew would enjoy the news. I also asked them to create social media posts for everyone who had committed in solidarity to wear their shirts on the day of my transplant.

In that moment, surrounded by my family, my heart was so full. We traveled in my white S.U.V., emergency bag packed, with hope permeating the cabin on the drive to St. Luke's. Ice storm or not, we were on our way.

The day that began like any other ended as the day that would forever change my life—the day life gave me one more chance to live #Lemonadelife.

Yusef's Hope and Disappointment with the Failed Kidney Transplant

When we pulled up to St. Luke's that icy New Year's night, I felt like I was stepping into the promise I'd waited so long for. We made it early, 8:00 p.m., a good thirty minutes before I was supposed to be there. I walked into that emergency room carrying not just my overnight bag, but nearly five years of hope, suffering, exhaustion, and prayers whispered on dialysis chairs.

They greeted me with warmth and a wheelchair, then handed me a small, soft pillow shaped like a kidney—a keepsake to commemorate what I thought would be the day I reclaimed my freedom. That simple gesture struck me. After so many nights lying awake, wondering if I'd ever get this chance, I finally held something that said, "Today is the day."

Tamika, my wife, switched into warrior mode the minute they wheeled me back for prep. She'd been by my side through too many hospital stays, too many botched sticks by shaky-handed phlebotomists who struggled to find my veins. Her voice was steady, strong, when she told them we needed someone with real experience this time—not another round of trial and error on my arms. I could see the tension in her shoulders melt a little when they rolled in a specialist with an infrared vein finder—a little mercy, at last. That vein finder has become a great stress reliever over the years.

Once the IV was placed, we had a few quiet moments together— Tamika and I—just sitting there, trying to believe this was really happening. They started the anesthesia meds. That's the last thing I remember.

Sometime in the early hours of January 2, around 2:00 a.m., the transplant surgery began. They told me later that the procedure ran long because of unexpected challenges—things my sedated body would never feel but that I'd carry the weight of later. A Foley catheter was placed, and the new kidney nestled into my right lower abdomen. Just like that, a new piece of me was stitched into place.

When I woke up, I woke up fighting. My first memory after the fog of sedation was panic! I came to with a feeling of suffocation. I couldn't breathe! It was like my lungs were wrapped in plastic. Instinct took over before reason could. I remember the tangle of arms trying to hold me down, which heightened my anxiety. Nurses were yelling, machines were beeping, but all I knew was that I needed the breathing tube out. It came out, pulled by my own hands and raw survival instinct. That was my first taste of the anxious battle ahead.

The pain was excruciating—the deep, throbbing soreness in my belly where they'd cut me open, the port jammed in my neck, the catheter a constant reminder that my body wasn't fully my own yet. They told me that before I could leave the ICU, I'd have to pass a bowel movement. That became my singular goal. I had to get through the fog of pain and focus on that one task, so I could get out of that room where fear and trauma clung to the walls like stale air.

When I finally did, they wheeled me to the kidney transplant recovery wing. Only my fight wasn't over—not by a long shot. They said the new kidney wasn't "awake" yet. It needed time to adjust, to learn to do what it was made to do. So, I had to sit through three more dialysis sessions, each one a cruel reminder that freedom was still just out of reach.

For eight long days, I walked the transplant floor in my gown and slippers, catheter in tow, pushing myself one foot in front of the other because they told me walking would help. The first time around, the unit felt impossible. Then twice. Then four laps. I was determined. Maybe if I kept moving, this kidney would wake up and catch up with me.

They made me climb stairs before I could be discharged. Each step was like a whispered prayer that this fight would be worth it. Every day, I watched the bag attached to my Foley for signs that my urine was clearing. Bloody red became pale pink, then a faint yellow. It felt like hope, drop by drop.

Inside that hospital room, I was isolated from the world, my immune system intentionally shut down so my body wouldn't see my new kidney as an invader. Tamika was my only visitor, my lifeline. Our friends and family, our #Lemonadelife supporters, flooded

Facebook with messages and prayers. They knew they couldn't visit, but they stayed with us in every word they posted. Anthony Smith, my old friend and classmate from Washington High, found a way to drop off food for my family—a small act of love that meant so much.

One photo I posted showed the port in my neck. My friend and nurse, Megan Randle, spotted the wrong caps on it right away—the non-sterile orange ones instead of the sterile green ones. Her quick message likely saved me from an infection I couldn't afford. I learned then that surviving a transplant wasn't just about the surgery; it was about every tiny detail that could make or break you in recovery.

Years later, as a nursing professor, Megan invited me to speak to her nursing classes and answer questions regarding my transplant journey. Her students asked thoughtful questions, and several approached me afterward, tears streaming down their faces, deeply moved by what they heard. Coincidentally, my daughter worked at the same college in the admissions office.

When I finally walked out of that hospital, the road ahead was still steep. Twice a week, I was back for post-transplant clinics, labs, and constant monitoring. My arms were bruised from so many needles, blood drawn repeatedly. Each visit felt like a checkpoint: Is this kidney working? Will my body accept it?

Unfortunately, the complications came anyway—rejection scares, hospitalizations, biopsies that showed no rejection, yet the treatments came just the same. I caught infections: E. coli, BK virus, and the shadow of CMV, which sparked bitter disagreements between doctors who couldn't agree on what was real. A wound vac at home, ports and PIC lines, and endless drips of antibiotics did little to fix what was broken.

After nearly a year of fighting—pills, prayers, tears, and a stubborn spirit—I sat in that clinic in December 2018 and heard the words I dreaded: I was officially back in Stage IV kidney failure. End-stage renal disease again.

The kidney I'd waited for, prayed for, fought for—the one that was supposed to free me from the dialysis chair—never truly took root. What started as my #Lemonadelife day felt, in the end, like waking up from a beautiful dream to find the storm still raging.

Even so, I remind myself: I had a chance. I tasted the hope. And though it slipped through my fingers, I'm still here. Still standing. Still squeezing these lemons for all they're worth.

Discrimination in the Medical Field and the Overdose of Tacrolimus

In 2018, I was forty-six years old, creeping up on forty-seven— nearly half a century of living with my skin being read like a warning label by strangers, bosses, neighbors, and now, doctors. I could run my fingers along the timeline of my life and trace all the ways racism had branded me. Pulled over and harassed for driving while Black. Falsely accused. Passed over for jobs I was overqualified for. Called "nigger" out loud far too many times and countless times silently. Still, nothing prepared me for how racism would show up in the place I was most vulnerable—a hospital room.

I thought of my parents, born in 1949, and all they'd endured as young Black souls in the heat of the civil rights era. My father loved to tell us stories from his college days—the time he and his classmates were nearly gunned down by highway patrol officers for daring to protest on campus, their only crime being Black and unbowed. I thought of my mother's family history—how some of my grandmother's kin fled to Coffeyville, Kansas, carrying the smoke and blood of the Tulsa Massacre in their bones. My maternal grandfather grew up in a dusty little railroad town called Havana, Kansas, scarred by racial violence just like Tulsa. He joined the military, found his way to Coffeyville, and met my grandmother. That's where they raised my mother and her siblings before moving to Kansas City, Kansas.

Then there was my paternal grandfather, an orphan boy in segregated New York, growing up in the only Black orphanage because even children without parents weren't safe from the color line. Each generation carried its wounds forward, hoping the next would bleed less. And I— standing four generations removed—once believed my daughters would be the ones to finally outrun this curse.

Yet as my kidneys failed, America's old ghosts found new ways to haunt my family. I watched my girls navigate a world that shouted "progress" from its billboards. Meanwhile, Black bodies—Trayvon Martin, Michael Brown, Eric Garner, Alton Sterling, Sandra Bland, George Floyd—fell to the pavement, reminding us how fragile Black life still is in America: "land of the free and home of the brave." Raising two daughters in that climate meant sleepless nights, eyes constantly scanning for the next threat. I needed to survive my illness for them—to protect them with every breath in my body.

So, when I sat in the exam room, fighting for my life after my transplant, the last place I expected racism to creep in was from behind the white coats and polite smiles of my care team. Shockingly, it did.

I remember asking my post-transplant nephrologist why they'd waited so long to test whether I was truly allergic to penicillin. His answer stopped me cold: "Clinically, African Americans have a stronger immune system. We were waiting for your superhuman immune system to kick in."

Superhuman? The word felt like acid in my ears. In that moment, I wasn't a patient, a father, or a husband fighting to stay alive. I was just another Black body, a stereotype in a lab coat's mind. I said to that doctor right then and there, "Treat me like a human being, not by the color of my skin." However, the damage was already done.

When I dug through my lab results, I discovered another layer of injustice: the Caucasian eGFR and the African American eGFR, side by side. Numbers deciding who gets a transplant, who gets to live, who keeps waiting. At first, I shrugged it off. We get asked about our race on every form, every application, every intake sheet. You almost grow numb to it.

When I learned that the National Kidney Foundation and the American Society of Nephrology, in 2021, finally recommended removing the race modifier—when I learned that Black patients like me had been systematically denied transplants because of inflated numbers—my heart sank. How many lives were lost? How many families were forced to watch their loved ones wither away on dialysis, all because an outdated, biased formula told them we were not "qualified"?

By the time they finally tested my supposed penicillin allergy, I'd spent ten months fighting infections—E. coli, BK virus, even a scare with CMV—while my doctors kept trusting my "superhuman" immune system to do what their prescriptions should have done. When the test results came back, the truth was clear: I wasn't allergic to penicillin at all. If they'd checked sooner, maybe the infections wouldn't have carved so deeply into my body's chance at healing. Maybe my kidney wouldn't have been forced to fight so hard to do its job.

Incredibly, it didn't end there. Tacrolimus, the anti-rejection medication I was prescribed, carries a dangerous side effect: kidney scarring. My care team should have known that. They should have monitored it like a hawk, but they didn't. They let the side effects creep in, unchecked, until my new kidney—the one I'd hoped would free me—was sixty percent scarred. Unusable. Dead weight inside me.

I remember sitting in that closed-door meeting at St. Luke's with my nephrologist and the post-transplant director, feeling the hollow weight of their halfhearted apology. They offered me a so-called "backroom deal"—a promise to put me back on the transplant waitlist in "inactive" status. They never admitted the truth outright. Never called it what it was: neglect, bias, the fatal arrogance of seeing my Blackness before they saw my humanity.

As they talked, I felt my spirit sink under the weight of the words I'd waited so long to hear—not an admission of guilt, but the final nail in the coffin of a dream. I'd fought a war for a new life and lost to the same old enemy my father, my grandparents, my ancestors had fought before me: systemic racism disguised in polite conversation and medical degrees.

I retreated from that room bewildered, disgusted, and broken. How could I explain to my family that after all the needles, the scars, the hope, I was headed for an inevitable return to dialysis? Back to lymphedema. Back to swelling, infections, and days blurred by pain and exhaustion. Back to being tethered to a machine for survival.

I spent so many nights asking myself the same question: Why me? But deep down, I knew it wasn't just me. It was my father who was almost shot for daring to demand equality. My ancestors, who were forced to flee Tulsa's bombs and flames. The countless Black bodies who never even made it onto the transplant list because the numbers lied about their worth.

This was the cost of racism in the system—not just the loss of a kidney, but the slow theft of hope. That said, I still wake every day, determined to live my #Lemonadelife despite the sour taste it leaves behind.

Chapter V

Unraveling the Racism

Exploration of Institutional Racism in Healthcare

Since my own painful and discouraging experiences in the healthcare system—especially the bitter disappointment of an unsuccessful kidney transplant—I have found myself digging deeper into the roots of why people like me, people who look like me, so often find ourselves on the losing end of the medical spectrum.

At every turn, I am met with the hard truth: America's healthcare system has long been infected by a quiet, insidious disease—institutional racism. This is not simply an opinion formed from my own trials, but a fact long recognized by scholars, health workers, and even government reports.

The Institute of Medicine's landmark 2003 report, *Unequal Treatment: Confronting Racial and Ethnic Disparities in Healthcare*, declared plainly: "Evidence of racial and ethnic disparities in healthcare is, with few exceptions, remarkably consistent across a range of illnesses and healthcare services."

Think about that—consistent across the board. These are not isolated incidents; they are woven into the very fabric of our medical institutions.

Long before this, the U.S. Department of Health and Human Services' *Report of the Secretary's Task Force on Black and Minority Health* (1985), commonly known as the Heckler Report—the first federal report to comprehensively document health disparities—exposed that Black Americans suffered an excess of deaths compared to whites that was "as high as 60,000 per year." The report boldly concluded: "The mortality rate among African Americans was substantially higher for eight of the ten leading causes of death."

Yet, despite decades of such revelations, the gap remains stubbornly wide. Harriet A. Washington, in her groundbreaking book *Medical Apartheid: The Dark History of Medical Experimentation on Black Americans from Colonial Times to the Present* (2007), laid bare the horrific history that built this divide. She writes: "Black Americans were more frequently deceived, coerced, and forced into experiments, a pattern that continues to this day in more subtle but equally insidious ways."

What's worse is that these biases are not only historical relics. They are alive and well in our hospitals and clinics. *Just Medicine* by Dayna Bowen Matthew (2018) shines light on how implicit bias poisons treatment decisions, often unconsciously. She writes: "Physicians do not have to intend to harm their patients in order for implicit bias to have a deadly effect."

This isn't just theory. It is lived reality for people like me, my family, and my community. The recent 2024 report, *Revealing Disparities: Health Care Workers' Observations of Discrimination Against Patients* by the Commonwealth Fund and the African American Research Collaborative, reveals the gut-wrenching truth: "Nearly half of Black health care workers report witnessing discrimination against Black patients in the past year alone."

So, when I sit in an exam room—fighting to keep my dignity while the person in the white coat assumes things about me they'd never assume about someone else—it's not paranoia. It's history. It's policy. It's bias passed down like an heirloom no one wants, but too few are willing to bury.

It's high time—past time—for American healthcare to finally rid itself of these systemic biases, these stereotypes that rob people like me of our right to live, to heal, to hope. Our health is not expendable. Our bodies are not experiments. Our lives are not footnotes in medical textbooks. We are human beings. We deserve care unmarred by racism. And that fight, to tear the rot out by the roots, starts by naming the truth out loud.

Yusef's Encounters with Bias and Prejudice

How disappointing, how soul-crushing, that after centuries of so-called progress, I find myself in a cold, sterile exam room in 2018, asking the same question my ancestors must have whispered in the dark: when will we be treated as fully human?

To truly understand how the shadows of the past follow me into every clinic, every lab, every prescription slip, you must see the bitter path that brought us here. Look at how the centuries line up, a grim timeline of stolen humanity—a history that still lives in my veins, my scars, and the eyes of my daughters:

1619: The first African human beings are brought in chains to the English colony of Virginia.

Mid-17th Century: Laws are created to codify Black enslaved human beings as property, making bondage hereditary.

1662: Virginia law dictates that a child's status—free or enslaved—is determined by the mother's condition.

1775–1783: Some Black Africans fight for the British, others for American independence, dying for a freedom they are denied.

1777: Vermont abolishes slavery in its constitution; other Northern states follow with slow, gradual steps.

1787: The "3/5ths Compromise" is written into the U.S. Constitution, declaring my ancestors to be three-fifths of a person for representation and taxation—a fraction that still echoes in the treatment of Black lives today.

1793: Eli Whitney's cotton gin explodes the demand for enslaved labor in the Southern states.

1808: The importation of Africans for enslavement is outlawed, yet domestic slave breeding thrives.

1831: Nat Turner's rebellion sparks such terror that white slaveholders turn his skin into lampshades and preserve his testicles in formaldehyde, trophies of their dominion over Black flesh. Recipes circulate for the consumption of Black bodies, proof that dehumanization runs deeper than any law could pretend to undo.

1850s: The Fugitive Slave Act was passed, forcing free states to return escaped enslaved people to their owners. Slave patrols are formed—the blueprint for what would become America's local police.

1857: The Dred Scott decision rules that no Black person, enslaved or free, can be an American citizen.

1861–1865: The Civil War erupts: slavery is its undeniable root.

1863: The Emancipation Proclamation is issued, freeing enslaved people in Confederate territory—on paper, anyway.

1865: The Civil War ends. The 13th Amendment abolishes slavery; the 14th grants citizenship to all born here, but the dream of equality is stillborn.

1877: Reconstruction ends. White supremacist groups rise, and segregation becomes law across the South.

20th Century: America says it knows slavery was wrong, but its actions remain tangled in contradiction, passing down injustice like a family heirloom.

And now, here I am—a Black man with scars from dialysis needles, a failed kidney transplant, and a heart that refuses to stop asking why. Why, after all that history, must I still sit in a doctor's office and wonder if they truly see me as deserving of life?

In my post-transplant clinic, the echoes of slavery whisper every time a nurse questions my "compliance." They linger when a physician's tone suggests that my suffering must somehow be my own doing—that my body is suspect, lazy, unworthy. I feel the 3/5ths compromise burning at the back of my throat every time my pain is brushed aside or my story second-guessed.

It is not paranoia. It is not imagined. It is centuries of proof.

The Institute of Medicine's report, *Unequal Treatment: Confronting Racial and Ethnic Disparities in Healthcare* (2003), lays it bare: "Evidence of racial and ethnic disparities in healthcare is, with few exceptions, remarkably consistent across a range of illnesses and healthcare services."

The Heckler Report—formally titled *Report of the Secretary's Task Force on Black and Minority Health* (1985)—admitted what too many still refuse to name: "The mortality rate among African Americans was substantially higher for eight of the ten leading causes of death."

The brilliant Harriet A. reminds us in *Medical Apartheid: The Dark History of Medical Experimentation on Black Americans from Colonial Times to the Present* (2007): "Black Americans were more frequently deceived, coerced, and forced into experiments, a pattern that continues to this day in more subtle but equally insidious ways."

Dayna Bowen Matthew's *Just Medicine: A Cure for Racial Inequality in American Health Care* (2018) explains how bias hides in plain sight: "Patients of color are more likely to have their symptoms underestimated, their pain undertreated, and their questions left unanswered. All because of biases physicians may not even realize they hold."

The Commonwealth Fund & AARC report, *Revealing Disparities: Health Care Workers' Observations of Discrimination Against Patients* (2024), shows us how this legacy lives on: "Nearly half of Black health care workers report witnessing discrimination against Black patients in the past year alone."

So, when I sit there—my veins raw from needles, my mind exhausted from the mental gymnastics of wondering if I am being judged, dismissed, or discarded—I carry this timeline with me. I carry my daughters' faces, bright and unbroken, hoping they will never feel the weight of being three-fifths of anything. I carry the ghost of Nat Turner, who died for the idea that we are whole and holy—not commodities for profit, experiments for study, or statistics to be ignored.

It is high time—past time—for American healthcare to rip this poison out at the root. To bury the myth that racism ended with a single amendment or a single election. To do what centuries of laws and empty promises could not: honor our humanity without conditions, disclaimers, or fractions.

My story is just one in a sea of millions, but I speak it out loud because silence has never set us free. Let the record show that I was here, that I fought to be seen, and that I refuse to leave my children a world where they must shrink themselves to fit the measure of a broken system. We are whole. We have always been whole. And we deserve to be treated that way—in every hospital, every clinic, every moment we entrust our bodies to a system that owes us nothing less than the truth: *Black lives are not 3/5ths. We are everything!*

Chapter VI

The Allergy Oversight

Inability to Test for Allergies Due to Racial Assumptions

Tacrolimus—an immunosuppressant so many kidney transplant recipients rely on to keep their new organ alive—carries a hidden blade. While its purpose is to protect the kidney from rejection, it comes with a well-known risk: nephrotoxicity. In other words, Tacrolimus can slowly poison the very kidney it is meant to protect, causing chronic damage known as interstitial fibrosis and tubular atrophy (IF/TA)—what I came to know all too well as kidney scarring.

This isn't new science. It's not a mystery. Research has long confirmed this risk. Studies published in journals like the American Journal of Transplantation and Transplantation Reviews show that African American transplant recipients face an even steeper climb. Genetic differences, especially in the CYP3A5 enzyme, mean African Americans often metabolize Tacrolimus faster, requiring higher doses to hit the target therapeutic range (Staatz & Tett, 2004; McNicholas et al., 2020).

However, this "higher dose" has a double edge: while it might suppress the immune system enough to prevent rejection, it also raises the risk of kidney toxicity and scarring. Research in Transplantation Reviews (Kwun et al., 2021) found that elevated Tacrolimus levels strongly correlate with increased kidney fibrosis and atrophy, especially when dosing is not closely tailored to each patient's genetics.

In my case? No one looked at me as an individual with a unique genetic profile. No one tested me for my CYP3A5 status. They never asked if I might be at higher risk for Tacrolimus-induced scarring. They never paused to question if my "higher-than-normal" dose was slowly carving away at my new kidney's lifespan.

Not once in any conversation or medical note was Tacrolimus flagged as the likely cause of the scarring that ate away my new kidney until it was too late. In just ten short months after my transplant, my new kidney was ruined. Over 60 percent was scarred all because of an oversight born of an old, persistent belief: that an African American male must have a "superhuman" immune system.

So here we are again. Racially differentiated treatment without the individualized care to match it. Here was an opportunity for my medical team to proceed with caution, to test, to monitor, to adjust, but they didn't. The catastrophic result of this assumption was a new kidney, gifted to me with hope, that failed before it ever had a chance.

Consequences of Not Addressing Potential Complications

When the damage was finally undeniable, I had to stop taking Tacrolimus altogether, though removing Tacrolimus didn't mean I was free. It just meant trading one chain for another. We had a new plan: a different immunosuppressant, Belatacept (Nulojix).

Unlike Tacrolimus pills I could take at home, Belatacept required me to report to an infusion center every 28 days, to sit in a recliner chair for an hour or more while an IV dripped medicine into my veins. It was an eerie echo of dialysis: the same chair, the same sterile rooms, the same feeling of being tied down. The freedom I thought I'd gained from dialysis was once again held hostage by a schedule.

This 28-day clock came with only three days of wiggle room—three days early or three days late—before my body risked rejecting the kidney. Spontaneity disappeared. Trips out of town had to be mapped carefully around infusion centers. Missing an infusion wasn't an option. Some days, I'd leave that chair feeling hollowed out, like life had been drained from me. Whether it was physical or mental, it always hit me physically.

Doctor appointments, dental work, and labs all had to orbit around this rigid cycle. When COVID-19 forced the whole country into lockdown, people were frantic about isolation and masks. But for me, quarantine was nothing new. I'd been living it since January 2018, forced to limit contact, mask up, and avoid crowds merely to stay alive.

When my doctor finally cleared me to travel on March 15, 2018, I was overjoyed. I got to take a flight to a company-sponsored resort in Tucson, Arizona—finally, a taste of normalcy. Sadly, two days into the trip, I came down with something—vomiting, exhausted, fighting to hold on while my wife, Tamika, stayed by my side. She should have been out celebrating an award she'd won at work, but there she was, caring for me instead. I urged her to enjoy the festivities. Yet because of who she is, she stayed.

We made the most of our final day in an unexpectedly cold Arizona. I soaked in the sun, the freedom, the air that didn't smell like hospitals. Even at that moment, the shadow of the next infusion hung over me. The leash was waiting back home.

Then came the final gut punch. During one of my annual transplant evaluations, I learned that my time on Belatacept had an expiration date too. Studies have shown (Kidney International Reports, 2019) that over time, patients can develop antibodies against Belatacept, rendering it ineffective. Once that happens, you must stop it forever.

I asked my transplant team what my options would be when that day comes. The answer? Go back to Tacrolimus, back to the drug that robbed me of my kidney the first time.

I felt like I'd been punched in the gut by my own future. I asked the obvious question: "Why would I take a drug that destroyed my kidney?"

Their answer? "We'll just have to monitor it more closely this time."

I was appalled. I thought, *Why didn't you monitor it closely the first time?* But that question doesn't matter anymore. The oversight, the assumptions, and the consequences can't be undone.

The Real Cost

The true cost of bias and blanket assumptions in medicine is clear: dreams deferred, lives shortened, and families forced to watch loved ones suffer from avoidable errors.

For African American kidney recipients like me, individualized, race-conscious care isn't just about good medicine; it's a matter of survival. Careful genetic testing, thoughtful monitoring, and honest conversations shouldn't be special requests. They should be standard.

My fight isn't over. I'm still tethered to my 28-day leash at the time of this writing, still juggling the costs of someone else's oversight. Still telling this story so the next patient like me doesn't have to ask, "Why didn't you catch this sooner?"

This is my #Lemonadelife—finding hope in a system that was never built for people like me, and squeezing every drop of truth out of the bitterness they tried to make me swallow.

Chapter VII

Post-Transplant Complications

Yusef's Struggles with the Aftermath of a Failed Kidney Transplant

My struggles with the aftermath of my failed kidney transplant truly began to intensify on January 1, 2020. However, the reality is that my body and spirit had been fighting this uphill battle long before that date. That New Year's Day, I was still dealing with what I thought was just a lingering cold that I'd caught the week after Christmas. Yet as each day passed, my symptoms grew worse. No amount of rest, soup, or cough drops could shake it.

I did what I always did when something felt off: I asked my father to take me to the emergency room at St. Luke's—the hospital that had performed my kidney transplant, where all my records lived. I'd made it my habit to go there for anything serious because they knew my body's fragile, immunosuppressed state better than anyone else. I was checked in, examined, and eventually diagnosed with Influenza A. They sent me home with codeine cough syrup and instructions for over-the-counter medication, but even then, deep down, I felt this wasn't just the common flu.

Back then, none of us really understood that COVID-19 had already arrived on American shores months earlier. I can see now how my new immunosuppressed body was a wide-open door for any infection that came my way. It was the end of January before I started to feel better, but the world was about to feel much worse. By March, we were living in a full-blown pandemic. The entire nation was ordered to wear masks, quarantine, and avoid anyone who might be sick. Though for me, masks and social distancing weren't new. Ever since my transplant, that level of caution had been my everyday life—the hidden reality of living inside a body that could betray me at any moment.

St. Luke's reached out to me quickly when vaccines became available. They identified me as "high risk for COVID-19" and urged me to get my free vaccination in two parts, two weeks apart. I didn't hesitate. I knew how much I needed every defense I could get, and it was offered to Tamika too. While the nation was thrown into a panic over mask mandates and vaccines, I felt an eerie sense of familiarity. The news showed bodies piling up in hospitals, then in morgues, and eventually in refrigerated trucks when there was nowhere else to put them. Friends in New York called me with whispers of sickness, loved ones dying, some too afraid to speak it out loud. Celebrities we thought untouchable began to fall one by one.

It was haunting. Life in 2020 reminded me of life post-transplant: the masks, the quarantining, the weird shopping hours I'd already adopted to avoid crowds, the escape plans I'd mapped out in my mind if someone coughed too close. I pulled out the leftover masks from my transplant days. Suddenly, the rest of the world looked like me. Despite my caution, I still caught

COVID-19 at least four separate times. Each time, I survived. Each time, I endured the fear of passing it to Tamika and the girls. I remember the loneliness of isolating in my own home, unable to hold my wife's hand. Meanwhile, Tamika, who'd started her CNA certification program in fall 2019, was terrified to finish. Nightly news reports told of entire nursing homes dying with what felt like no end in sight.

In February 2020, I faced another blow. My feet and knees began to swell painfully, the skin red and hot to the touch. Each day, the pain grew more unbearable until I could no longer make it down the stairs to my room. I grabbed my walking cane for support, then a walker, and finally set up camp on our living room couch near the bathroom, just three feet away. That tiny distance felt like a mile. I lay there for three months, day and night, sleeping and eating on that couch, taking Tylenol like candy but never finding relief.

I'd bought tickets for a Valentine's Day concert to see our good friend Lee Langston perform—a date night with my wife—but the pain made walking impossible. Instead, I sent Naqari to go with Tamika, hoping they'd enjoy what I couldn't. I tried to convince myself it was arthritis, but I was wrong. I hobbled to an orthopedic doctor, begging for knee shots. They gave them to me, but the pain never let up.

Back at St. Luke's, they ran labs and found my uric acid levels were dangerously high. My kidneys could no longer filter out toxins, and I had developed gout. The medication that could help could only be taken once a flare-up subsided. When the attacks are unrelenting, that relief never comes fast enough.

I remember the second week of June so vividly. The swelling began to ease, but not before I'd endured months where even standing up from my recliner to touch my feet to the floor brought tears to my eyes. It was one of the worst pains I'd ever known, aside from the relentless cramps during dialysis. My prayer life deepened in those days. I prayed for my own relief and, when it didn't come, I prayed for others. A friend of mine, Morris Letcher, had pancreatitis. He then suffered a stroke and fell into a coma for months. His sister Sonja Letcher secretly updated me, and I prayed for him daily. When my own pain wouldn't lift, I hoped my prayers would find him instead. He survived but was forever changed—a cruel reminder that sometimes survival comes at a price.

As I tried to adjust, I met with a dietitian, hoping to lose weight and control my diabetes. I learned that my diet—red meat, processed foods, turkey, seafood, and even mushrooms—was fueling my gout attacks. So, I switched to chicken and fish. Then my new rheumatologist prescribed allopurinol once the flare-ups calmed down.

Meanwhile, my old nemesis, lymphedema, returned. I'll never forget how, in the eight days I spent recovering from my transplant, I celebrated that my legs no longer needed compression socks. By 2020, the swelling was back with a vengeance. My legs were so swollen that walking was painful, sometimes impossible. The years of wearing compression garments had curved my big toenails inward, making them ingrown and infected.

Every attempt I made to return to my old workout routine was thwarted by gout, swelling, fatigue, and pain. One after another, they fell like dominoes.

Even before the pandemic, in late 2018, my body was sending distress signals. I'd feel overwhelming fatigue out of nowhere. Just walking from my car to the clinic door would leave me breathless and desperate to sit down. By March, I was driving to St. Luke's Infusion Center every 28 days for my Belatacept IV infusions, hoping to hold off my body's rejection of the kidney. I remember one visit clearly. My mother was in the hospital. She, too, suffered kidney failure. After my infusion, I drove from Missouri to Overland Park Regional to see her. When I got there, my phone rang. It was the transplant clinic: "Mr. Harris, we need you to come back.

Your hemoglobin is at six. You may need a blood transfusion."

At the infusion center earlier, I overheard my name on a phone call. *Why didn't they just keep me there?* I thought, but I turned around and drove back. The dread I felt walking in those hospital hallways, my breath shallow, is something I won't forget. I got my first blood transfusion that day. As I lay back, I thought about Arthur Ashe, the tennis great who contracted HIV from a transfusion. Was it really safe now? By then, my exhaustion left no room for that fear to linger.

Later, I was referred to an oncologist. Sitting in a cancer clinic waiting room made my heart pound. Thankfully, my low hemoglobin wasn't cancer, but it was one more complication with no apparent cause. My doctor explained my levels would never be normal again. No answers for the "why"—only more prescriptions and more monitoring.

While I fought to keep my body afloat, I had to face an unspoken truth: the odds had been stacked against me from the beginning. In America today, the average five-year kidney transplant survival rate for white patients is around 85 to 90 percent. For African American patients like me, that number drops to around 73 to 80 percent. We're less likely to receive a transplant, more likely to lose it sooner, and more likely to die waiting. The reasons are layered: unequal access to follow-up care, bias in the system, and the daily stress of racism itself. All these pieces add up. They did for me too.

So, every lab result, every flare of pain in my knees and feet, every swollen leg, every mask I wore long before COVID made it mainstream—all of it was a fight not just with my own body but with a system that has never treated people who look like me fairly.

Despite everything, I pressed on. The weight of gout, lymphedema, diabetes, hypertension, blindness in one eye, endless infusions, the fear of COVID-19, and a failed transplant that still haunts my body to this day—none of it has crushed my will to keep living. Because while my transplant failed me, I refuse to let my spirit fail too. I carry and share this story not just for me, but for the next person whose kidneys are failing, whose prayers feel unanswered, whose fight feels invisible.

Yusef's Mental Challenges with the Traumatic Experience of a Failed Kidney Transplant

So often, when we're battling something physical, the instinct is to throw every ounce of energy into fixing our body. However, the truth is, our minds can quietly break down long before we ever find a cure. Throughout every setback I've shared, underneath all the swelling, the needles, the tubes, and the failed promises of healing, there was a heavy mental burden I carried alone for too long.

I remember so clearly how it felt to be disappointed, overwhelmed, full of dread, and no one seemed to notice the toll that was taking on my mind. One of the nurses, during a routine visit, finally pulled me aside, spoke to me about being overwhelmed, and asked how I was feeling mentally. After explaining how bewildered, overwhelmed, and overstimulated I was, she referred me to a psychiatrist. I'll never forget her kind, patient demeanor as I poured out my worries about whether I'd ever be able to work again, whether my mind could keep up with all the medications and appointments and diagnoses, and whether my spirit could hold steady under the constant weight of things never going as planned.

Before my transplant failed, when I was still working, I was already well-versed in mental gymnastics. As a Black man in America, I'd been practicing that balancing act my whole life. It was normal for me to multitask, not just at work but also in how I had to manage people's perceptions of me. I knew I had to work twice as hard for the same paycheck as my white counterparts. I knew that if I wanted to provide for my family, I couldn't let the daily inequities wear me down on the outside, even as they chewed at me from within.

Even the simple act of driving to work came with its own mental calculations. From the moment I pulled out of my driveway, I had to run through the script every Black boy in America gets handed down: Don't look like a threat. Keep your head on a swivel. Make no sudden moves if you get pulled over, especially if the officer is white.

I remember driving to dialysis one morning at 5 a.m. in 2015, not long after Walter Scott, an innocent Black man, was shot in the back and killed by police. A young, nervous white cop pulled me over on a pitch-black road with no one around to witness whatever might happen. I knew I hadn't been speeding. I used cruise control religiously to remove any excuse for a stop.

I would often hear my grandfather, Rev. Alfred Treece Sr.'s words in my head: "If you're on time, you're late." So, I was always early. Yet there I was, stopped on a dark road with the officer's hand hovering over his gun.

His flashlight blinded me as he asked for my license and registration. I asked for permission before reaching for the glovebox. My hands were locked on the wheel at ten and two—a grown man in his truck, silently replaying the worst-case scenario. I wasn't new to being pulled over, but this time, dread crept in where indignation used to live. That same posture we're taught to keep on the road, we carry into the corporate world too. Soften your tone. Don't come off too confident. Don't make people feel small with your competence.

I remember one performance review at Sprint where my Caucasian female supervisor told me she wanted to share feedback from my peers, managers, and supervisors. She told me I was "ominous" in meetings—that my presence, my preparedness, and my questions intimidated my superiors. I'd spent my life being the kid in the Talented and Gifted program, the one who thought outside the box, the one who didn't just meet expectations but shattered them. Yet in those rooms, my brilliance wasn't seen as an asset. It was a threat. So, I learned to dim my light, pick my moments, and soften my posture to get the merit raise that would help me take care of my family.

Not every boss made me feel that way. Don Newsom, a Caucasian at Sprint, saw my worth. He respected me and made sure I was compensated well for it. My merit reviews under him were some of the best I'd ever had. That validation meant more than money; it gave my mind a little oxygen.

Before him, Mike Bragg, another Caucasian manager, pulled me aside to lead the offshoring project that would save Sprint millions. My wife still remembers the pride in Mike's voice when he told her, "Your husband is such an asset to this company."

My Caucasian female director, Karen Sage, fought tooth and nail with the benefits office to make sure I got the durable medical equipment I needed to keep working on the offshoring project while blind in my left eye. The benefits department said it wasn't covered, and I would have to pay out of pocket for the equipment. Karen wrote a one-page letter detailing the millions of dollars I was singlehandedly saving the company and told both them and Human Resources that they *would* be paying for my equipment. Reading that letter and hearing her explain my value to the company was validation. These moments were precious mental fuel for a mind constantly under siege.

The truth is that my body paid the price for my mental acrobatics. I worked so hard proving my worth that I lost an eye, developed lymphedema that would never entirely go away, and spent nights awake worrying about whether my value would ever outweigh my exhaustion. I single-handedly created training materials that offshored an entire help desk, but I hadn't even earned a million dollars in my ten-year career while saving the company millions. The mental arithmetic of that eats at you.

Too often, in the Black community, we're told we don't need therapy—that it makes us weak, that we're "crazy," or that we can't handle our business. But the day I walked into my therapist's office, I finally saw what I'd needed all along. He looked like me. He had a wife and daughter like me.

He understood me. He explained my anxiety clinically, telling me how my brain's chemicals misfired when the trauma caught up to me. He told me my coping skills were strong but gave me tools for the days when they weren't enough.

I remember when my good friend Megan Randle, who was teaching nursing at KCKCC, called me in 2023. She asked me to share my transplant story with her class. For the first time, I stood at a podium, mask off, and spoke my pain out loud. I laid out my time-line from memory, took questions, and felt the weight of students leaning in to understand what I had survived. I remember leaving that room feeling a flicker of self-worth I hadn't felt in a long time. Megan asked me back every semester. Each time, I gave the truth of my scars to a roomful of future nurses, so they'd see their patients as human beings, not just bodies to fix or medicate.

Before my last presentation to Megan's class, she asked me to write everything down chronologically so it would flow better and leave time for more questions. During my time as a corporate trainer, I joined clubs such as Sprint Masters and Toastmasters to sharpen my public-speaking skills. Those groups helped me cut filler words, orga-nize my thoughts, and get comfortable speaking to a room. When I finally wrote out my timeline for Megan's students, it forced me to focus on the details. In the middle of that presentation, as I walked them through my story, I realized what was at the root of my anxi-ety—that moment in the ICU when I woke up and pulled my own breathing tube out.

Telling that story triggered me right there in class. I saw it all over again—the dark, the suffocation, the panic. A female student began sobbing, unable to contain how unfair it all was. I tried to console her during class and afterward, but that moment showed me how deeply my mental wounds had been buried just to survive.

I spoke to a lawyer in 2024 about my transplant and all its failures. I did this after discussing it with my therapist. The thought had never occurred to me. I contacted a few lawyers provided to me by my friend Alonzo Jamison's wife, Colleen. One of the city's malpractice law firms was on the phone. I told her the reason for the call and began discussing my medical condition. After a myriad of questions from the paralegal, the last question was, "When was your transplant?" I explained it was January 1, 2018. "Oh, I'm so sorry!" She told me I had missed the statute of limitations for a malpractice suit by two years in both the State of Missouri and Kansas.

I sat there, devastated. How could I have known to fight when I'd been so busy trying to live?

My therapist told me plainly, "The system failed you. Completely." Then he added, "You need to write this book." It was the only justice left.

It was my friend Lee Langston who first handed me a blank journal at a bookstore, telling me, "Man, write this down." I did for a while, but life and surgeries and a failed fistula revision that forced me to face more disability paperwork than my trembling hand could handle overwhelmed me. I was terrified my benefits would vanish if I was no longer deemed disabled by the constantly rotating disability coordinators. When I told my therapist how the memories crushed me every time I tried to write, he said, "You have to. It'll heal you." So, I used what I knew best—technology—and created an outline for #Lemonadelife.

Now, therapy has changed everything. It's helped me make sense of the scars no one can see. It helped me show up better for my wife, who's endured so much alongside me. It helped me hear my daughters when they tell me I'm the best dad they could ask for, even when I don't feel that way. It helped me sit still and breathe through the memories.

If I could tell anyone anything, it's this: you must tend to your mind as fiercely as you tend to your body. Don't wait until you're shattered to pick up the pieces. It's 2025 now. I'm a month into my second time on dialysis, but I'm finally writing #Lemonadelife. I'm closer to my goal weight, so I can get back on the transplant list. I'm living proof that when life gives you lemons, you find a way to squeeze them into something sweet for yourself and for the ones who come after you.

When life gives you lemons... Live #Lemonadelife.

Chapter VIII

Fighting Back with Advocacy

Advocacy—The Lifeline We All Need

Advocacy is not just important—it's vital. In today's healthcare system, every patient deserves an advocate, especially in moments of crisis, confusion, or vulnerability. Whether it's a trusted relative, friend, or yourself, having someone speak up on your behalf could mean the difference between life and death.

Let's start with the obvious: if you're seeking medical care, it's because something isn't right. Yet you're often expected to absorb a flood of medical information, make rapid decisions, and consent to serious procedures, all while you're physically and mentally overwhelmed. That's not just unreasonable—it's dangerous.

Unfortunately, this is the reality in a healthcare system that often prioritizes efficiency and billing over individualized care. According to the CDC, six in ten adults in the United States have a chronic disease, and four in ten have two or more. That's a staggering portion of our population struggling with serious health concerns, yet the system treats patients like data points instead of human beings.

So how do we fight back? We advocate. Here's what I've learned through lived experience:

1. You're Sick—You Need Support

When you're ill or in pain, your ability to comprehend, remember, and assess complex medical information is compromised. That's why having a loved one or advocate present matters. They can ask questions, push for clarity, and help ensure decisions aren't rushed. They can demand time to consider second opinions, research procedures, and fully understand diagnoses.

2. You Must Become Your Own Advocate

It's not just OK to question your care—it's necessary. Learn your condition. Understand your lab results. Know what medications are being prescribed and why. Research how these medications affect people of your racial or ethnic background. This knowledge is power, and it equips you to push back when something doesn't seem right.

3. Don't Be Afraid to Speak Up

If something feels off, say so. Ask questions. Challenge assumptions. The healthcare system is not infallible. Racial bias, systemic neglect, and miscommunication happen more often than we want to admit, and they're frequently deadly.

4. Advocate for Others

If you know someone in your family who's vulnerable—an elder, someone who's anxious around doctors, someone who's too sick to think clearly—volunteer to go with them. Sit in the room.

Take notes. Ask the questions they can't.

Let me illustrate how powerful and necessary this can be with two stories from my own life.

My Aunt's Silent Struggle

When my Aunt Rosie Horn fell into a coma, I visited her every day. I knew she was diabetic, so I asked the nurses about her blood sugar. It was dangerously high, but they were only giving her a mere three units of insulin. I asked to speak to the endocrinologist, but because I wasn't an immediate family member, they ignored my request.

Hospitals often give the bare minimum while charging the maximum. Without someone pushing for proper care, my aunt suffered unnecessarily. Though she eventually came out of her coma and went to rehab, she passed away shortly afterward. I can't help but believe that stronger advocacy could have changed the outcome.

Saving My Mother's Life

When my mother was hospitalized with heart and breathing issues, I was there every day. Her swelling was increasing rapidly, and after they removed a fluid output monitor due to discomfort, they stopped tracking her condition altogether. I asked a doctor about the swelling and risk of pneumonia. His response? "She probably won't get pneumonia."

That wasn't good enough for me.

I pressed further. The nurse admitted they weren't tracking her fluid levels anymore. Only after my questioning did the doctor order them to resume tracking. That alone was disturbing, but it got worse.

One morning, after briefly leaving the hospital for a follow-up of my own, my father and I returned to find my mother's bed empty. No call, no explanation, even though we had asked to be contacted before procedures. She had been scheduled for a heart procedure without notifying her primary caregivers, who were my father and me. Even worse, when she voiced that she couldn't breathe during the procedure, the doctors ignored her. A nurse had to step in and advocate for my mother, who couldn't breathe in the position she was being forced into.

Later, when she was moved to CICU, I asked the medical team why they hadn't considered dialysis, given that my mother had a functioning fistula and was a kidney transplant patient. The doctor looked stunned and said, "That's a great idea! I never thought of that." He even jokingly said, "We're going to have to start calling you Dr. Yusef."

I wasn't laughing. I was livid!

They gave her two dialysis treatments, tapped each lung, and, miraculously, she began to recover. The swelling went down. She could breathe. She was alive. But if I hadn't spoken up, if I hadn't insisted, if I hadn't known what to ask, that might not have been the case.

Trauma on the Operating Table

Even my own surgeries weren't immune from negligence. During my first vitrectomy surgery, I was supposed to be sedated. Instead, I came to, feeling the surgeons cutting my eye. I had to force myself to speak through the sedation and tell them I was awake and in pain.

I will never forget that moment. It's a scar just like the physical ones left behind from failed fistula revisions and previous surgeries.

Speaking Up for Systemic Change

Today, one way I fight back is by sharing my story. Thanks to my friend Megan, I had the opportunity to speak with nursing students about real-world healthcare and the critical role they play in it. My story puts a face to the consequences of systemic neglect. It's not just about symptoms and procedures. It's about human lives.

Racial bias is not a footnote in healthcare—it's a headline. Yet it's not being taught in classrooms or addressed in curricula. That must change. Every healthcare worker, new or seasoned, should be trained to identify and eliminate racial bias from their practice.

We can't fix what we won't face.

Know Your Rights

Whether you're checking into a clinic or an emergency room, ask to speak with the hospital's patient advocate. Request a copy of your patient's rights. Know them. Learn them. And demand that they be honored. Education is your armor in a broken system.

We live in a profoundly unhealthy country. According to the National Health Interview Survey, over 133 million Americans—more than 40 percent of the population—live with at least one chronic disease. The numbers are rising, not falling. Hospitals are overburdened, undertrained in bias awareness, and focused far too much on profit over people.

The parking lots are full for a reason: America is sick. Too often, we lose our lives to things that the right care, the right questions, and the right advocacy could have prevented.

We are not powerless. We can educate ourselves. We can speak up. We can save lives, starting with our own.

Networks That Challenge Discrimination

When life gives you lemons… Live #Lemonadelife.

I created #Lemonadelife as more than a catchy phrase—it became a spiritual and practical mantra for surviving the battle against kidney failure. At first, it was a vision: to build something that could support other kidney transplant patients through monetary assistance, education, and advocacy tools. As my own health and financial security unraveled due to systemic failures, the mission evolved.

I became a living case study, an unwilling sacrifice, exposing the racial inequities and indifference built into our healthcare system. Through each painful setback, I began documenting and sharing the reality: Black and Brown patients, the underinsured, and those simply lacking advocates often suffer not from their conditions alone, but from neglect, ignorance, and bias.

Without asking, I became a guide for others. Friends and family began reaching out for advice, support, and direction as they navigated their own healthcare crises. While I never set out to become an advocate or healthcare educator, people watched closely—sometimes silently—as I overcame challenge after challenge and still stood.

People often ask me, "How do you do it?"

Let me tell you plainly: It's my faith not just in myself but in the Most High.

I believe in the one many call Jesus Christ, or in Hebrew, Yeshua Ha'Mashiach. It is my faith in G-D, my Elohim, that has carried me through trauma, surgeries, misdiagnoses, hospitalizations, abandonment, and yes, survival.

I know this may not reflect everyone's belief system. There are many faiths, many interpretations of spiritual truth, and some who walk in no religion at all. But this is my truth. It is my witness. It is what gave me strength, resilience, and mental clarity to face an unjust healthcare system and not just survive but fight for others too.

As it says in the scriptures:

Acts 2:38 (KJV)

"Then Peter said unto them, Repent, and be baptized every one of you in the name of Jesus Christ for the remission of sins, and ye shall receive the gift of the Holy Ghost."

Ma`asei 2:38 (TS2009)

"And Kĕpha said to them, 'Repent, and let each one of you be immersed in the Name of עשוהי Messiah for the forgiveness of sins. And you shall receive the gift of the Set-apart Spirit."

I share this to affirm that even when systems fail, my faith does not. It is my cornerstone—the unshakable foundation I stand on when everything else collapses.

Building a Collective Fight Against Healthcare Discrimination

As I continue to walk this path, battling injustices in healthcare and beyond, I never forget to look for ways to uplift others while also taking care of myself. This fight isn't one person's burden to carry alone. Thankfully, there are growing networks and organizations across the U.S. and globally working to dismantle racism, classism, and neglect in medical care.

If you or someone you love is navigating this system, feeling voiceless or unseen, here are impactful organizations and resources actively fighting for equity in healthcare:

Active Networks Challenging Discrimination in Healthcare

1. **The National Health Law Program (NHeLP)**
   The National Health Law Program advocates for the rights of underserved populations to access quality healthcare. They address discrimination, Medicaid protection, and racial health disparities.
   • www.healthlaw.org

2. **The Center for Health Equity (CDC)**
   The Center for Health Equity works to reduce health disparities through systemic change in public health and social policy, primarily affecting communities of color.
   • CDC Health Equity

3. **The National Medical Association (NMA)**
   The National Medical Association, the largest and oldest national organization representing African American physicians and patients in the U.S., works to eliminate disparities and advance equitable health outcomes.
   • www.nmanet.org

4. **Black Women's Health Imperative (BWHI)**
   The Black Women's Health Imperative focuses on the health and wellness of Black women and girls, challenging systemic neglect through policy, education, and advocacy.
   • www.bwhi.org

5. **Patient Advocate Foundation (PAF)**

The Patient Advocate Foundation helps patients navigate insurance denials, medical billing, and discrimination in care. They are especially useful for low-income patients facing barriers.

- www.patientadvocate.org

6. **Race Forward / Healthcare Equity Action Network**

Race Forward helps institutions confront systemic racism, offering tools for inclusive, anti-racist health policy reforms.

- www.raceforward.org

3. **Health Leads USA**

Health Leads USA focuses on addressing social determinants of health, such as housing, food access, and income security as part of patient care.

- www.healthleadsusa.org

4. **Campaign for Anti-Racism in Medicine (CAIR-MED)**

CAIR-MED is a growing grassroots movement of students and professionals pushing medical schools to deconstruct racist curriculum and practices.

- CAIR-MED Instagram

Final Thought: Turn Your Pain into Purpose

This journey has taught me that survival is more than a miracle. It's a mission. When systems are broken, when medical care is flawed, and when the world tells you to be quiet and compliant, you must find your voice. Sometimes, it means becoming the advocate you wish you had.

#Lemonadelife is not just mine. It belongs to anyone who has had to turn trauma into purpose, pain into power, and survival into service.

Because in the end, when life gives you lemons, you don't just make lemonade. *You Live #Lemonadelife.*

Chapter IX

Legal Battles and Activism

Yusef's Journey to Seek Justice for Medical Malpractice

In 2019, after receiving guidance from a patient advocate at a different medical facility, I followed the appropriate protocol. I then contacted the patient advocate at St. Luke's Hospital to file a formal complaint. I sought clarity on why my kidney transplant had failed and what the next steps were to obtain another transplant. This was especially urgent given that, in October 2018, the nephrologist on my transplant team had verbally assured me that I would have a chance for another transplant. That assurance was based on the fact that my newly transplanted kidney never functioned above Stage IV due to scarring.

When I approached the patient advocate, I was told, "I can't take your complaint," and was redirected to someone else. She escorted me to the post-transplant clinic—the same place I had been visiting weekly since being approved for a kidney transplant. This redirection was not just dismissive; it bypassed the hospital's established process for formal patient complaints and stripped me of the opportunity to have my case fairly reviewed. It was a negligent act that prevented accountability and obscured the systemic failures in my care.

In a private meeting room at the clinic, I sat with the nephrologist and the director of the kidney transplant clinic. They gave me an informal, undocumented explanation. Tacrolimus, the anti-rejection drug they prescribed, was the cause of the transplant failure. While they initially blamed viral infections for the scarring, they ultimately admitted Tacrolimus was responsible. I asked why, given the drug's known side effects, they didn't err on the side of caution. The response was chilling: "We just didn't figure it out in ten months."

I left the meeting stunned and heartbroken. Although the transplant team claimed they would try to get me listed again for a second transplant, they now explained that the United Network for Organ Sharing (UNOS) would not permit a new transplant unless my current kidney was fully inoperable. The strategy was to let me remain with a poorly functioning kidney until I inevitably needed dialysis again. Only then, according to the team, could I be relisted—and even then, in inactive status.

For eight months, the lead nephrologist told me he was working on getting me another transplant right away, always dangling the promise of rectifying the kidney's failure to respond as expected. It was a blow to any optimism I had held on to through the excruciating recovery I faced every day.

I walked away from that meeting without legal counsel, without advocacy, and without hope. I didn't know my rights. I was never educated on the Patient Bill of Rights, either before or after my transplant. Emotionally and physically drained, I was overwhelmed by a flood of lab work, doctor's visits, and the relentless toll of managing my failing health. Defeated, I spent the rest of 2019 wondering when dialysis would return and if I'd ever get a second chance at life. My mental health deteriorated as I questioned everything I had endured.

Not once during this time did the hospital acknowledge fault or conduct a full review of its protocols, prescriptions, or treatment decisions that I was made privy to. Instead, blame was quietly and subtly shifted onto me, my body, my biology, my Black skin. There was no transparency, no apology, and certainly no accountability. My kidney was allowed to deteriorate, leaving more than 60 percent irreparably scarred.

Then, in early 2020, the world changed as the COVID-19 pandemic emerged. I navigated that frightening era with a compromised immune system and Stage IV kidney failure, praying that the virus wouldn't push my already fragile kidney past the point of no return.

It wasn't until 2022, four years after my transplant, that multiple healthcare professionals and a therapist asked a pivotal question: Have you ever considered filing a malpractice lawsuit?

Until then, I hadn't even thought of it. I had been too busy trying to survive.

I consulted a medical malpractice attorney that year, armed with thorough documentation and a clear timeline of my experience. The attorney listened intently, then asked one simple but life-altering question: "When did you have your kidney transplant?"

I responded, "January 1, 2018."

His reply hit me like a freight train: "I'm so sorry. You would have needed to file your case by 2020. The statute of limitations in both Kansas and Missouri is two years. It sounds like you have a strong case, but legally, there's nothing we can do now. We've been fighting to change this law because many patients don't even realize they've been victims of malpractice until it's too late."

My breath left my body. I felt gutted. The anguish, the rage, the helplessness—all resurfaced with devastating force. I had been led down a path that ended in legal invisibility. My family and I had invested so much emotionally and financially in my recovery, only to be left without options. My health was crumbling, and my rights had been swept under the rug by an unforgiving legal clock I wasn't even aware of.

Even more heartbreakingly, the very hospital that had pledged to save my life had failed me at every critical juncture. I was left with a failing kidney, more than fifty daily medications, weight gain that disqualified me from the transplant list, and new health challenges that seemed to multiply with time.

Later in 2022, I was officially removed from the transplant waitlist due to my weight—a cruel irony, considering the weight gain was caused by a kidney that could no longer filter toxins. At a follow-up evaluation, I asked why I was being removed from the list if I wasn't even on dialysis yet, which was supposedly the condition for relisting. The physician confirmed my suspicion: even if I had met the weight requirement, I still wouldn't have been eligible because I wasn't yet on dialysis.

When I pushed further, they quickly shifted focus to a small ulcer near the fistula in my left arm, booking an appointment with a vascular surgeon. I agreed to the revision out of fear that the ulcer could become life-threatening. That surgery in 2022 was another episode of sedation and seemed to resolve the issue for two years.

However, in 2024, the growth bulge returned in my left arm. Since I knew my kidney health was declining, I went back to the same surgeon who had done my earlier revision. Trying to be proactive with my health because I knew I would need a working fistula for dialysis, we devised a plan to revise my current left arm fistula with an AV graft. In November 2024, I scheduled the surgery. I left the operating room with thirty staples, an inoperable and clotted fistula, and ongoing hand tremors—a new complication from a system that had already failed me so profoundly.

Statute of Limitations for Medical Malpractice

Kansas:
Under Kansas law (Kansas Statutes Annotated § 60-513), medical malpractice claims must be filed within two years from the date of the act or when the injury becomes reasonably ascertainable. However, no claim may be filed more than four years after the date of the malpractice itself, regardless of discovery.

Missouri:
Under Missouri law (Revised Statutes of Missouri § 516.105), medical malpractice claims must be filed within two years from the date of the negligent act or when the injury is discovered or should have been discovered. Certain exceptions apply for foreign objects, failure to inform of test results, and minors. However, no claim may be filed more than ten years after the date of the malpractice itself, regardless of discovery.

As a resident of Kansas and having my medical services performed in Missouri, I had no additional resources to pursue a medical malpractice claim. These laws need to be reviewed and amended to ensure that medical patients who suffer from malpractice have legal recourse. The legislation is written to favor the medical institution, limit patient protection, and, in some cases, prohibit it.

Broader Implications: Exposing Systemic Bias in Healthcare

My experience isn't just my own; it's a symptom of a deeper, systemic issue. There's a pervasive, outdated belief that Black bodies have a "superhuman" resistance to illness. Yet, at St. Luke's, there was no DNA analysis or scientific basis to support that notion: no lab results measuring my genetic resilience, just assumptions rooted in skin color.

"Where is the study that says what percentage of my African American DNA possesses the superhuman healing factor?" I questioned. "Where is the study that shows, based upon your percentage of African American heritage, you have the corresponding percentage of human healing factor in your immune system?" The answer: there isn't one.

It's well documented that racial and ethnic biases plague medical research. One review found that over half of U.S. clinical trials between 2000 and 2020 did not report enrollment data by race and ethnicity, and when they did, White participants were significantly overrepresented.

The report *Racial and Ethnic Disparities in Access to Medical Advancements and Technologies*

by Nambi Ndugga, Drishti Pillai, and Samantha Artiga (published Feb 22, 2024) bluntly states: "People of color are often underrepresented in clinical trials. A study found that over half of U.S. trials between 2000 and 2020 didn't report enrollment data by race and ethnicity, and among those that did, White people were overrepresented."

Meanwhile, the integrity of medical research has been called into question. Epidemiologist John Ioannidis famously asserted that "as much as 90 percent of the published medical information that doctors rely on is flawed," citing issues like bias, low-quality design, and publication pressure. This staggering claim highlights how systemic errors, not skin color, often drive health disparities.

These failures aren't abstract. They affect real lives, including mine. Protocols like estimated glomerular filtration rate (EGFR), which guide transplant decisions, have historically used race as a biological marker, even though race is a social construct—not a biological proxy. This bias resulted in me being under-prioritized for transplant eligibility, masked as medical reasoning.

Systemic racism extends beyond diagnostic criteria. It permeates the doctor's office. Implicit biases built into outdated training and flawed research lead to misdiagnoses, under-treatment, and poor outcomes. The pandemic only magnified these issues. People of color experienced a disproportionate burden—not because of genetics, but due to pre-existing conditions linked to structural inequality.

Our healthcare system is stretched thin. Overbooked physicians, interminable waiting rooms, and insufficient time for patient follow-up point to a fractured system. Even parking and valet shortages are indicators of a crisis. COVID-19 left permanent cracks in healthcare infrastructure, eroding trust and access, particularly for those with chronic conditions like mine.

Still, change is emerging. More researchers and advocacy groups are pushing for inclusive clinical trials and unbiased diagnostics, but progress is slow. Demographic misrepresentation, flawed methodologies, and underfunded bias-awareness programs keep turning hope into rhetoric.

In my case, racial bias wasn't just a factor. It was a linchpin in the negligence I experienced. The medical team focused on my biology and skin color, not the clearly evident side effects of a prescribed medication. That choice shattered my health, financial stability, and trust in medicine.

I survived, but so many more continue to suffer. Countless families face financial ruin from medical debt, and lives are cut short by undiagnosed or mismanaged conditions. Justice is not just personal—it's fundamental.

What Must Change

- Demand transparency in clinical trials: all studies should report comprehensive demographic data.
- Eliminate race-based medical metrics, such as EGFR adjustments, and replace them with individualized biomarkers.
- Sanction mandatory bias training for all healthcare professionals.
- Ensure equitable access and empathy-based care, not rushed appointments driven by quotas.

My story is proof that systemic failures cause harm, but also that one voice can spark awareness. It's time to build a healthcare system grounded in human dignity, scientific rigor, and justice.

Chapter X

Hope and Resilience

Yusef's Perseverance and Determination in the Face of Adversity

Perseverance, in its purest form, means continuing forward—holding fast to a goal despite opposition, pain, or setbacks. It's that unrelenting spirit that refuses to be broken, no matter how fierce the storm. Determination is its close companion: a focused will, shaped by reflection, trial, and deep internal resolve.

When I look in the mirror, I don't just see my reflection; I see perseverance and determination staring back at me. If you've read this far, I hope you've seen how these two themes have woven themselves into every part of my story, from childhood to now. They didn't just appear overnight. They were cultivated over years of struggle, healing, failure, and growth. From the beginning, I believed—whether in success or in failure—that I had the capacity to press forward.

When I gave my life back to G-D, I began to see perseverance and determination through a new lens, through the truth of Scripture. I clung to the promise found in Philippians 4:13 (KJV):

"I can do all things through Christ which strengtheneth me."

Or as it's rendered in the TS2009 translation:

"I have strength to do all, through Messiah who empowers me."

As a child and teenager, I was curious and determined to understand how things worked. I would take apart electronics just to see the inner workings. At first, I'd forget where each screw went, but over time, I learned to take things apart methodically. It wasn't just trial and error. It was perseverance in action. Every failure was a lesson, and every success a quiet victory.

But that same confidence didn't come easily in my spiritual walk. Faith, I found, was different. Hebrews 11:1 (KJV) says:

"Now faith is the substance of things hoped for, the evidence of things not seen."

In the TS2009 version:

"And belief is the substance of what is expected, the proof of what is not seen."

When I first read this, it dawned on me that we already practice faith every day without realizing it. When you sit in a chair, you trust it will hold your weight. When you start your car, you expect it to turn on. That's faith—simple, unconscious belief.

Though when it comes to people, faith becomes more complicated. I used to carry strong faith in others, expecting the best. While some fulfilled that hope, others deeply disappointed me. Over time, I found myself lowering expectations to protect my heart. A quote I once read, often attributed to Bob Marley, struck a chord:

"The truth is, everyone is going to hurt you. You just got to find the ones worth suffering for."

I revisited this quote after my vitrectomy surgery. I returned to it during challenging chapters in my marriage and family life. Once again, it echoed through me after my kidney transplant. Life, health, relationships—they all forced me to reexamine where I placed my faith.

We're conditioned to believe that doctors have all the answers. That they can fix what's broken. Yet the reality is they didn't create us. They don't hold the blueprint of our bodies and souls. Believers understand that the true healer, the Great Physician, is Yahshua Ha'Mashiach—Jesus the Messiah.

Scripture tells us He healed the sick, raised the dead, gave sight to the blind, and restored the broken. But beyond physical healing,

He offered spiritual restoration—healing the deepest wounds of the human soul, washing away sin, and offering renewal through the Holy Spirit.

While I know not everyone believes this, I can only speak my truth: my strength, my perseverance, and my survival are rooted in my faith in Yahshua.

I don't force anyone to believe what I believe. But when people ask how I survived what I've been through—how I've endured pain, loss, and mistreatment—I give all glory to G-D, my Elohim, through His Son Yahshua.

"I can do all things THROUGH Christ which strengthens me."

Some may challenge that and ask, "If you believe in healing, why are you still suffering?" However, those questions don't take the entire picture into account. They don't recall the story of Job, or the three Hebrew boys who faced the fiery furnace, or Paul's thorn that was never removed. Yet Paul wrote in 2 Corinthians 12:9:

"My grace is sufficient for thee: for my strength is made perfect in weakness."

My life isn't over. I still believe G-D can completely heal me if it's His will. Even if He doesn't, like the Hebrew boys in Daniel 3:18, I choose to trust Him regardless:

"But if not, be it known… we will not serve your gods…"

At one of my lowest moments, during a difficult therapy session, my therapist said, "You are not the problem. The healthcare system has failed you completely." That broke something open for me. I realized I had to let go of misplaced trust in people and systems. I needed to put my full faith in G-D, but I also needed to take action.

Faith without works is dead.

So, I educated myself about my diagnoses, medications, and procedures. I became my own advocate, ensuring the same mistakes wouldn't happen again. I found strength in knowledge, in speaking up, and in sharing my story. I push forward not only for myself but for others, so they might suffer less.

Maybe someone reading this will become an advocate for their loved one. Perhaps someone will be inspired to challenge the system, to demand better. And maybe, when everything else seems lost, they'll find hope through faith, through perseverance, through the quiet truth that G-D is still able.

Together, we can demand change. Together, we can become the light in someone's darkest hour. So, when human hands fall short, I pray we always remember there is One who never fails.

The Impact of Yusef's Story on the Community and the Support of #Lemonadelife

My #Lemonadelife community has been nothing short of a lifeline for both my family and me. Their support has lifted us emotionally, spiritually, and yes, even financially, in some of our darkest hours.

When I first received my diagnosis of kidney failure, I was in the middle of publishing my first book, *OMG! My GOD, My GOD*. The weight of that news was overwhelming. I had so many unanswered questions, so much fear, but I still had a dream to finish and a purpose to fulfill. Around then, my longtime friend Rodney McNeal and I had a candid conversation. He encouraged me to share my story publicly, to let people in. Up until that moment, I had been private about my health struggles, caught between fear, pride, and uncertainty. His words planted a seed.

That seed was nourished by the wise counsel of Mrs. Patricia Hamilton, the mother of my dear friend Christopher Hamilton. She reminded me that disability wasn't a handout. It was a benefit I had earned through years of hard work. Her message, delivered with care, broke through the shame I carried. I cried tears of pride and release. I had been approved for disability before, after a failed vitrectomy, but chose to work again when I got hired at the Federal Reserve in 2010. I was trying to do what was best for my growing family, unaware that the system wasn't built to explain the process clearly or compassionately. Now, I was being called to choose myself, my health, my life.

Rodney's encouragement helped me break the silence. He worked in the medical field, and our friendship ran deep. He was the only one who could've convinced me to go public with my condition, and so I did. As I released my first book, I also began navigating the foreign and frightening waters of end-stage renal disease.

With the realization that I'd need financial help to afford medications while on disability and later dialysis, I turned to HelpHOPELive, a 501(c)(3) organization that allowed me to raise funds transparently. My dear friend and classmate, Michelle Wilson Knobel, wasted no time in creating my fundraising page. Still, something was missing—a rallying cry. A slogan that captured my will to live, my need to fight, and my hope for healing.

After tossing around ideas with Michelle, the phrase came to me:

When life gives you lemons... Live #Lemonadelife.

It wasn't just a clever twist on an old saying. It was a declaration: I was choosing to live, not just survive, and now I needed to show people what that looked like.

That's when my creative spirit was reawakened. I met with Michelle and my childhood friend Thomas McIntosh III, an incredibly gifted DJ whose talents I'd admired since we were teenagers at Skateland. There, we expressed ourselves through music, style, and dance. Now, decades later, we were coming together again—not for fun, but for a mission. Thomas offered to lend his DJ skills to a benefit event, and Michelle stepped in to organize it. Together, we envisioned a joyful gathering, a celebration of community rising to help a friend in need.

Yet I still needed a visual identity, something tangible to represent this movement. A couple of years later, Thomas personally introduced me to Donald "Scribe" Ross, a gifted graffiti and graphic artist whose work could be seen throughout the city. Scribe was transforming environments at Children's Mercy Hospital, helping kids escape into color and imagination amid their battles with illness. We met at "Soulful Sundays," where DJs like Thomas and Bryan "DJ Ataxic" Fisk played healing sets of soul, R&B, and hip-hop. That place was a sanctuary. I told Scribe about my vision, and he listened deeply. He asked me to email a description of what I needed, and then he went to work.

What he created blew me away!

My vision—lemons, hope, fight, purpose—came to life in a logo that instantly captured everything #Lemonadelife stood for. When I offered to pay him, he refused. His generosity moved me beyond words. That logo, now on the cover of this book, is a symbol of a community bound together not by shared health struggles, but by shared humanity.

With shirts printed through Custom Ink and later perfected with help from my church brother Eric Wells and Brown Bear Printing in Leavenworth, Kansas, the movement began to take on a life of its own. People started wearing their shirts in support of me. Then something extraordinary happened. People began connecting because of it. Total strangers would see each other wearing a #Lemonadelife shirt and instantly share a story, a memory, or encouragement.

During the time leading up to my transplant, something even deeper happened. My friend Bryan "DJ Ataxic" Fisk, who had once lifted my spirits through music along with Thomas McIntosh at Soulful Sundays, fell ill with a heart condition. I visited him in the hospital, brought my wife to sing for him, and got to know his wife, Trinessa. What started as a visit turned into a lifelong friendship. Despite their own challenges, they gave generously to support my journey. That's the kind of love that #Lemonadelife brought into my life.

In 2016, friends, family, and even people I'd never met came together for a benefit event filled with music, laughter, and generosity. Auction items poured in—memorabilia from NFL players Greg Hill, Marcus Allen, Lake Dawson, Cam Newton, and Victor Cruz. Tennis champion Venus Williams sent signed tennis balls and a signed tennis racquet, courtesy of my good friend and brother Carlos Flemming. Michael Brantley took the signed tennis ball and racquet, along with a photo of Venus Williams, and created a shadowbox frame for them with a material that looked like court grass. I received gifts and assistance from local heroes who believed in the cause. Signed jerseys, tennis rackets, gift cards, hotel stays, and catered food turned a fundraiser into a community festival of love.

I reconnected with old friends like LaDale Beason, who welcomed me into his circle of DJ brothers, including Joseph Straws III, Jeron Slater, and Derrick Garlington. As we bonded over music and mixes on "Mix Mondays," they bought shirts, posted to social media, and spread the message. LaDale's clients at his salon started asking about the movement, and soon, even more strangers became family.

As the shirts traveled, so did the message about kidney health, transplantation, and the power of community. From NFL legends like Marcus Allen and Bobby Bell to the Kansas City Royals' World Championship team, support kept pouring in. Perhaps one of the most poetic full-circle moments came when James Anderson—the man who inspired me to become a barber— provided his signature drink, James' Lemonade, for my #Lemonadelife event. How perfect is that?

The event was DJ'd by Thomas and Bryan, and the keynote speaker was my brother and dear friend, Todd "T.J." Johnson. T.J. had inspired me before I ever coined #Lemonadelife with his own mantra, #NoZer0Days, as he battled POEMS syndrome and worked his way back to walking. That night, watching him step up to the podium, cane in hand, as he addressed the crowd, I was in awe. He was once my inspiration, and now he was helping me inspire others.

Of course, I cannot speak of this journey without honoring my dear friend Randall "Randy" Chestnut. Randy was one of the most selfless, kind-hearted men I've ever known. We bonded in high school over his quiet act of protection, warning me about a rumor a scorned ex-girlfriend was spreading about me before we were even friends.

Later in life, as we both faced health battles, we leaned on each other with phone calls full of prayers, jokes, and encouragement. Randy showed up to my event, sick but smiling. Not long after, he visited me in the hospital. He prayed over me, filling the room with peace and power. I will never forget the calm that came over me as he hugged me and said, "I love you more, Brother."

He passed away in July 2020, a few months before his birthday in October. I miss him dearly. Rest in Eternal Peace, Randy.

Through all the hospital visits, financial struggles, fundraising, and setbacks, one thing remained constant: my people showed up. My family, my friends, my community, and complete strangers walked beside me, lifting me higher when I felt I couldn't take another step.

#Lemonadelife became more than a motto. It became a movement. A testament to what hope, love, and faith in each other can build, even in the face of a failing body.

Even now, as I face new challenges, I carry their love with me every day.

Chapter XI

Conclusion

Yusef's Ongoing Battle and the Broader Call for Healthcare Equality

Today, I continue to fight a battle—one that never truly ended when I left the hospital. The nightmare that followed my kidney transplant lingers in my body, my spirit, and my daily life.

I know now that my transplant didn't offer me the long, high-quality life I hoped for. Not because of fate, but because of an overdose of Tacrolimus and the unspoken, deeply rooted racial bias in modern medicine. The truth cuts deeper than any scalpel.

It's traumatic. It's exhausting. Most of all, it's infuriating.

There were countless moments when I could've given up. Moments when despair tried to swallow me whole. Though somehow, some way, I always chose to fight. Looking back, I know it wasn't just grit or willpower that carried me. It was the grace of G-D, my family's unshakable love, and the collective support of a community that believed in me even when I couldn't see the light ahead.

In early 2025, something shifted. For the first time, I began to see what others had been seeing in me all along. I was in a training class, and after it ended, my instructor, Steve Scott—who was a stranger to my story—asked about what I was going through. As I spoke, listing the challenges one by one, I saw his face shift. His eyes widened. His jaw dropped. He was stunned. He politely commented, "I didn't know." In that moment, I saw my own life reflected back at me, and it shook me to my core.

When I walked out to the car where Tamika was waiting, tears quietly streamed down my cheeks. I looked at her and said, "I finally saw what everyone else was seeing." I had heard it for years—family and friends telling me I was their hero, their inspiration. They looked up to me and couldn't imagine how I kept going. My answer was always the same: G-D. Because the strength I've needed, especially in the darkest moments, has never come from me alone. It's always been spiritual.

Still, I told Tamika through those tears, "I can't afford to feel the feelings they're feeling. I have to keep fighting. If I don't... I won't survive."

That moment in March revealed a crack in my armor. The warrior was growing tired. I was emotionally fatigued. Just as I began to feel the weight of it all threaten to take me down, G-D, in His infinite mercy, gave me a divine reminder to keep living.

On April 9, in the quiet early hours of the morning, my grandson Shakur Ahmed Harris was born—the first boy in a line of grandbabies. When I held him—fresh, warm, and perfect— something in me reignited. His soft curls, radiant skin, and grey eyes peering up at me, brand new to this world, breathed fresh life into me. In that moment, I wasn't just a survivor. I was alive. I had something new to fight for. A new future worth protecting.

Despite tremors in my left hand from a failed fistula revision just months earlier, I held Shakur steady. I admired his tiny frame, marveling at his presence. Then I went home to prepare for another surgery. My left arm, the same one that had faithfully carried me through nearly five years of dialysis, had finally given out. Now, I had to have a graft placed in my dominant right arm. It was something I didn't want, but something I needed. My creatinine numbers were rising. My kidney was declining. The return to dialysis was drawing near.

What followed was a series of complications, delays, and hospital stays that seemed endless. Each step revealed just how broken the healthcare system remains, especially for people like me—Black, vulnerable, and too often overlooked.

Through all of it—the trauma, the incompetence, the numbness in my hand that still hasn't gone away—I've kept walking forward. Not because it's been easy, but because survival demands it. I've spent nights in emergency rooms without beds, been misdiagnosed, dismissed, and ignored.

I've seen how quickly the system turns away from responsibility and how slowly it turns toward accountability. Yet, miraculously, I'm still here.

My story is a reminder: This fight isn't just mine. It's ours. We must dismantle the systems that allow this level of inequity to exist. The medical field must do better. Not tomorrow, today.

Through it all, I've chosen not to become bitter, but better. I've chosen not to be defined by what was taken from me, but by what I still must give. What I have is my story, my truth, my fire, and the hope that someone else reading these words will find the courage to keep going too.

Because *if life gives you lemons… Live #Lemonadelife.*

Yusef's Continuation of Inadequate Healthcare

From June 2 through June 6, 2025, I was admitted to Overland Park Regional Medical Center. After months of swelling, tingling, and numbness in my right arm, I had placed high hopes on Thursday's scheduled fistulagram with the very surgeon who had installed the graft. I was desperate for answers and some sense of closure.

That Tuesday, however, brought a mix of relief and chaos. I received my first dialysis treatment in seven years after the surgeon finally gave permission for the hospital to use my graft. It was Tamika's birthday, and while I wished we could be celebrating, we were instead sheltering together in a hospital hallway due to a tornado threat. Patients, nurses, and doctors huddled under fluorescent lights with doors closed tight, praying the storm would pass. It eventually did, but the chaos outside seemed to seep into the very walls.

Later that day, they moved me to a different wing, and things began to deteriorate. Staff response times dropped, and a noticeable lack of attentiveness emerged. Still, I had love around me. My oldest daughter, Naqari, on maternity leave, was by my side with my grandson, Shakur. I watched her with pride—my travel partner during AAU basketball days, now a mother herself. She placed Shakur on my chest, where he'd nap, just as he had dozens of times before. We had developed a bond in those early months, his small body resting on mine as we both drifted off in rhythm. Holding him reminded me of all I still had to live for.

Soon, more of my family arrived—my parents, my brother Omar, and my nieces Brooklyn and Morgan. It was a full-circle moment. I felt seen. I felt loved. I was finally mentally preparing for the Thursday procedure.

But then Thursday dawned, and with it came disappointment.

That morning, I was placed on NPO status at midnight, as required. I hadn't eaten in over twelve hours, but I wasn't hungry thanks to Mounjaro, which was paused and restarted several times during my surgeries. Just before noon, a staff member from the surgeon's office came into my room. The news hit me like a brick. The surgeon who placed my right arm AV graft had been called to another hospital for an emergency and would not be performing the procedure.

While I understand emergencies happen, this felt like yet another abandonment. I had consented, mentally and emotionally prepared, and was now being handed off again. I was asked to sign a new consent form for another surgeon and the radiology team to do the fistulagram. Resigned and weary, I agreed.

What followed was an all-too-familiar cascade of miscommunication and medical failure:

11:00 a.m. I was informed that Dr. Cameron had canceled the procedure.

12:00 p.m. No transport had come for me. I asked again.

1:00 p.m. The rounding physician said she'd look into the delay. She never returned.

2:00 p.m. I pressed the nurse call button again. They told me transport would arrive by 2:30 p.m.

2:35 p.m. I was finally taken down for the fistulagram.

4:00 p.m. I returned from the procedure with no clear answers. No one followed up.

I was offered a turkey sandwich I couldn't eat due to my gout, and when I requested a diabetic-friendly option, I was given a dry chicken breast on a bun, a cookie, and unsweetened iced tea. After nearly sixteen hours without food, this was insulting.

I was informed I would not receive dialysis that evening, despite being told otherwise.

The case manager, who admitted to being new, confessed she hadn't confirmed a dialysis chair as promised. I was told I couldn't be discharged until they found me a chair.

Then came Friday, June 6—a day I'll never forget for all the wrong reasons.

I was taken in for dialysis again. Two technicians attempted to cannulate my AV graft. They failed seven times. I begged them to stop after the fifth attempt, but the nephrology nurse practitioner pushed for two more—still, nothing.

Frustrated and in pain, I called the hospital's patient advocate line. I left a voicemail pleading for help. No one returned my call.

Out of desperation, I finally called Davita Wyandotte West. Their director answered and confirmed what no one at the hospital had told me: I had a chair waiting for me that Monday. With this knowledge, I was finally discharged late Friday afternoon, nearly twenty-four hours after my promised release.

That final day at the hospital felt like the embodiment of everything wrong with the system: miscommunication, apathy, and emotional fatigue. I noticed longer delays in nurse response, poor communication about test results, and inconsistency in the most basic elements of my care. It was as if once I stopped being a "priority" patient, I stopped being treated as a person altogether.

I left the hospital angry, in discomfort, and emotionally drained. It hit me that this was the same hospital that had nearly fumbled my mother's care just months earlier. Back then, I'd urged my father to contact the patient advocate, and we never received a return call. I wasn't expecting anything different this time.

However, surprisingly, I received a call on June 12. The patient advocate asked me to formally submit my complaints. I did, detailing every single failure, including a separate report about the sterility of the operating room where my graft was placed and my surgeon's repeated avoidance.

Their response? A sterile, templated letter. No accountability. No compassion. Just bureaucracy in a neatly formatted paragraph.

I also reported the situation to the state. I needed to believe that someone—somewhere—might care enough to do better.

That said, advocacy doesn't always come with victories. Sometimes it feels like screaming into a void. Once again, the theme of inadequate healthcare haunted me—loud and clear. I felt unheard. I felt unimportant. I felt dismissed.

This #Lemonadelife was starting to feel bitter, worn out, and tired. I was exhausted from having to be both the patient and the advocate, the survivor and the whistleblower. Even so, I kept moving forward because stopping was never an option.

Reflection on the Importance of Dismantling Inadequate Healthcare and Institutional Racism in Medicine

After continued phone calls and direct advocacy, I was finally assigned a permanent dialysis chair. On June 13, 2025, I returned to in-center dialysis. It wasn't ideal, but it was necessary. I asked for an earlier session—third shift was too taxing. They granted the request. So, on the morning of June 16, I set my alarm for 5:15 a.m. and prepared myself for the long, familiar road ahead.

That month marked a sobering realization. On June 24, during my infusion, my nurse noted a drastic drop in my weight. It hit me then just how much my body had been carrying and how much my failed transplant had physically burdened me. Nearly 80 pounds of excess fluid were now dissolving, treatment by treatment. Each session, I pushed for just a bit more fluid removal, safely challenging my body to reclaim itself. Clothes that once clung to me now hung loosely.

Even the newer ones didn't fit. I was shrinking under the weight of it all—literally and emotionally.

Then came July 22—another infusion appointment, another trial. My regular nurse was off, and my anxiety surged. I've had too many bad experiences with IVs, too many careless sticks, and avoidable mistakes. That day, I was blindsided again. I was informed they wouldn't be approving my anti-rejection medication. They were withholding the very drug meant to protect the kidney I had fought so hard to maintain.

I was stunned.

Frustrated.

Angry.

Here I was, less than a week from my 54th birthday, facing another health crisis again due to broken systems and bureaucratic neglect. It felt like déjà vu, and not the good kind. This #Lemonadelife was testing me once more.

Then, like a punch to the chest, I learned that Malcolm-Jamal Warner—Theo Huxtable, the childhood face of laughter and light—had passed away. He was just 54. The same age I was about to turn. His passing shook me deeply. It made me pause and ask the question I try not to dwell on: Would I make it to Tuesday?

I didn't have an answer, but I did have resolve.

I would push through. I had to push through. This #Lemonadelife, bitter as it sometimes tasted, was still mine to live.

Yet, after all I've experienced, I have to say what too many people in power continue to ignore: Healthcare must change. We need to return humanity to medicine.

We need medical professionals who treat every patient as if caring for their own mother, brother, or child. We need systems that don't just respond but listen. Systems that don't just document but care. Patients should never be bystanders in their own treatment. They must be partners, advocates, participants in the process—not ignored voices behind a chart.

That vein finder has become a great stress reliever for medical professionals with God complexes: humility is not a weakness. Admitting a mistake doesn't disqualify you; it dignifies the patient and makes you stronger. Too many doctors avoid accountability simply because their ego can't bear a bruise. But the scars you leave on patients run much deeper than pride.

It is also long past time for patients to be educated about their rights. Proactively. Thoroughly. We deserve to know what we are entitled to. We deserve legal support, advocacy, and justice when things go wrong—not silence, stonewalling, or gaslighting.

We must also acknowledge and dismantle the very real racial bias that exists in healthcare—bias that nearly cost me my life. It is not enough to call for equity. We must build it, demand it, and hold the system accountable when it fails because it will fail again unless we force it to change.

We must stop being reactive and become revolutionary in how we protect and preserve human life. We must amplify patients' voices. We must listen, not dismiss. We must shine light on dark corners. We must raise our expectations.

My story is not just a cautionary tale. It is a call to action.

No human being should endure the indignities I've suffered. No family should be traumatized by preventable errors. No one should have to fight this hard just to be treated with dignity.

Though until we center humanity—until we hold ourselves to the ideals that leaders like Dr. Martin Luther King Jr. reminded us of—we will continue to repeat the same sins of the past.

"We hold these truths to be self-evident, that all men are created equal."

That dream still demands action. That equality still requires a fight. So, I will keep telling the truth.

I will keep standing. I will keep living.

Because when life gives you lemons… Live #Lemonadelife.

Acknowledgments

Legacy #Lemonadelife Backer
Philanthropist Sandi Young

#Lemonadelifers
Mrs. Vicki Jennings
Mr. Raymond Smith
Dr. Tammy Huff-Johnson
Dr. Jayson Strickland
Mrs. Carmen Hill
Mrs. Frances Schaber-Brewer

Sweet & Strong
Mrs. Michelle Knobel
Mr. Brent Flournoy
Mrs. Angi Maher Scheele
Mr. Chris Foster
Mr. Cory Anderson
Mr. Robert Tribbett III
Ms. Carolyn Chestnut
Ms. Naqari Harris

Pitchers of Lemonade
Mr. Scott Price
Mr. & Mrs. Ellis and Joy Taylor
Pastor Charles Cofield
Mr. Dwayne James

Lemon Droppers
Mr. Luke Bobo
Ms. Joyjean Verner
Ms. Nicole Chestnut

Dear #LemonadeLife Family,

From the depths of my heart, thank you.

Every piece of #LemonadeLife apparel you've worn and every dollar you've given toward my medical journey has meant more than I can fully put into words. What may have felt like a simple purchase or a small donation to you has been a powerful reminder to me that I am not walking this road alone.

Your support has helped lift real burdens during a very real season of life. But beyond the financial help, you've given me something even greater — encouragement, strength, and the motivation to keep pushing forward with faith, purpose, and hope. Every shirt, every hoodie, every act of generosity tells a story: that "When life gives us lemons, we don't quit… we live #LemonadeLife."

Because of you, this journey has become more than a personal health challenge. It has grown into a movement of resilience, faith, advocacy, and love. You are part of that story now. You are part of the impact. And I carry your kindness with me into every doctor's visit, every recovery day, and every step toward the future.

Thank you for believing in me. Thank you for standing with me. Thank you for showing what community truly looks like.

With deep gratitude and love,

Yusef Harris
#LemonadeLife

For future apparel campaigns and donations please visit us at:
www.ilivelemonadelife.com

References

Centers for Disease Control and Prevention. "About Chronic Diseases." *Centers for Disease Control and Prevention.* Accessed December 11, 2025. https://www.cdc.gov/chronicdisease/about/index.htm.

Crais, Clifton, and Pamela Scully. *Sara Baartman and the Hottentot Venus: A Ghost Story and a Biography.* Princeton, NJ: Princeton University Press, 2009.

DeGruy, Joy. *Post Traumatic Slave Syndrome: America's Legacy of Enduring Injury and Healing.* Portland, OR: Uptone Press, 2005.

Diao, Jessica A., et al. "Race Correction in Clinical Algorithms." *New England Journal of Medicine* 383, no. 9 (2020): 875–882.

Eneanya, Nwamaka D., et al. "Reconsidering the Consequences of Using Race in Kidney Function Estimation." *New England Journal of Medicine* 383, no. 9 (2020): 874–882.

Hoenig, Melanie, and Martha Pavlakis. "Removing Bias from Devices and Diagnostics Can Save Lives." *Nature*, October 23, 2024. https://www.nature.com/articles/d41586-024-03410-5.

Johns Hopkins Medicine. "Johns Hopkins Health System Adopts Race-Free Kidney Function Equation." *News Release*, February 10, 2022. https://www.hopkinsmedicine.org/news/newsroom/

news-releases/2022/02/johns-hopkins-health-system-adopts-race-free-kidney-function-equation.

Jones, James H. *Bad Blood: The Tuskegee Syphilis Experiment*. New York: Free Press, 1981. Revised edition, 1993.

Kwun, J., and S. J. Knechtle. "Overcoming chronic rejection—can it be?" *Transplantation Reviews*, 2021.

McNicholas, B. A., et al. "Belatacept: A review in kidney transplantation." *Drugs*, 2020.

National Center for Chronic Disease Prevention and Health Promotion. "Chronic Diseases in America." *Centers for Disease Control and Prevention*. Accessed December 11, 2025. https://www.cdc.gov/chronicdisease/resources/publications/facts-and-stats/index.htm.

Organ Procurement and Transplantation Network (OPTN). *Two-Year Race-Neutral eGFR Calculations Monitoring Report*. November 4, 2024. https://optn.transplant.hrsa.gov/media/ksuigccc/data_report_minority_affairs_committee_20241104.pdf.

Skloot, Rebecca. *The Immortal Life of Henrietta Lacks*. New York: Crown Publishing Group, 2010.

Staatz, C. E., and S. E. Tett. "Clinical pharmacokinetics and pharmacodynamics of tacrolimus in solid organ transplantation." *Clinical Pharmacokinetics*, 2004.

University of Maryland Medical Center. "University of Maryland Medicine to Eliminate Race from Kidney Function Estimates." *News Release*, November 21, 2021. https://www.umms.org/ummc/news/2021/eliminate-race-from-kidney-estimates.

Vincenti, F., et al. "Development of anti-Belatacept antibodies and its clinical consequences." *Kidney International Reports*, 2019.

About the Author

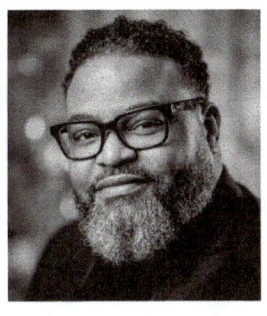 Yusef Harris is an author, advocate, and community builder whose work is rooted in empowering others through authentic storytelling and social awareness. His first book, OMG! My GOD, My GOD, released through B. Global Publishing, introduced him as a compelling new voice unafraid to challenge perspectives, elevate difficult conversations, and champion change.

With his second book, #LemonadeLife: The Book, Yusef expands that mission-offering a powerful, deeply personal account of his medical journey while confronting the systemic inequities that shape so many healthcare experiences. Through vulnerability, truth, and unwavering determination, he invites readers to transform pain into purpose and resilience.

A devoted father, husband, mentor, and lifelong community advocate, Yusef has spent decades investing in social activism, youth empowerment, and community development. He is committed to uplifting families, inspiring young people, and facilitating meaningful conversations about issues impacting the African American community.

Yusef studied Illustration at the University of Kansas, where he was actively involved in civil rights and social empowerment initiatives. Today, he continues educating and engaging audiences around the world through his Facebook community, "Black History Hosted by Yusef Harris."

Through his books, advocacy, and community engagement, Yusef Harris stands as a passionate voice for justice, healing, and transformation-reminding others that even in life's most difficult moments, something powerful and purposeful can be created.